Eat Often, Feel Great & Lose Weight

An Eating Plan to Curb Appetite and Prevent
Low Blood Sugar

Denise Dubé, RD, PDt, CNSD, BBA

All About Books Publishing • Montreal, Canada

**Eat Often, Feel Great & Lose Weight
An Eating Plan to Curb Appetite and
Prevent Low Blood-Sugar**
By Denise Dubé, RD, PDt, CNSD, BBA

Published by:
AAB (All About Books) Publishing
Post Office Box 563-A, Station H
Montreal QC, H3G 2L5 Canada
orders@aabpublishing.com
www.aabpublishing.com

ISBN, print edition   0-9781440-0-7
First Printing 2006
Printed in USA

SAN: 760-0259

CONTENTS

About the Author

Denise Dubé is a Registered Dietitian/Nutritionist, a member of the American Dietetic Association, and a Professional Dietitian, member of l'Ordre professionnel des diététistes du Québec.

She has counseled numerous patients and clients on weight loss over the past ten years in the USA and Canada, as a private consultant and as a hospital and medical clinic dietitian. She encountered many who described classical symptoms of hypoglycemia who later benefited from the diet recommendations described in this book. They lost weight without feeling very hungry or deprived.

Denise has a broad range of experiences in many areas of nutrition intervention including obesity, malnutrition as well as medical, surgical, cardiac, diabetic, renal, gastro-intestinal, pediatric, pulmonary and liver conditions. She has worked in intensive care, trauma and burn units and attained certification in nutrition support that is recognized by the American Society of Parenteral and Enteral Nutrition.

Her experience includes teaching nutrition classes to medical residents and interns. She now works as a home health dietitian where she counsels patients suffering from cancer, neurological and other conditions.

Would you go to an architect for legal advice? Would you ask a lawyer to build a house? Then why turn to anyone but a Registered Dietitian/Nutritionist for nutrition advice?

Acknowledgements

I am grateful to the many people who helped me along this endeavor. First and foremost, I thank my father, Raymond Dubé. He reminded me that the process of writing this book would be an enriching experience and "if the book sells, that's just a bonus."

Judith Kashul came to the rescue when other copy editing plans failed. Thanks to Hassan Arif for helping me patiently with my computer related questions, Hadi Halabi, my photographer and the friendly staff at Concordia Copies.

Warning—Disclaimer

INTRODUCTION

Are sudden feelings of intense hunger or cravings sabotaging your will power to lose excess body weight once and for all? Let's face it, no matter how well you try to follow a calorie-restricted diet, if it leaves you feeling hungry, you are not likely to stick with it long enough to reach your weight-loss goal.

Do friends, spouse or family members not understand how badly you feel when meals are delayed, and criticize you for not having enough "will power" to lose weight? It may be easy for them to say "stop eating so much" if they have very well balanced **insulin** and **glucagon** (hormones) levels enabling them to maintain blood sugar levels within normal range, even during extended periods of fasting. **Glucose**, the simplest form of **carbohydrate**, the preferred fuel of the body and the brain's indispensable fuel source, is in steady supply to them. They feel fine, therefore they can't understand why you can't eat what and when they do.

One day, a doctor from a family medical clinic where I worked entered my office to ask me which foods she could eat as midday snacks because she often gets sudden drops in energy and concentration, usually around 3 PM, accompanied with unshakable hunger. She asked "what can I eat to give me energy without gaining weight?" She stated that she found it difficult to shed extra pounds because when she went without a snack she tended to overeat at the next meal, yet she didn't want to consume extra calories by eating more often.

N.B: Text written in bold is defined in the Glossary

I gave her tips on certain food options along with physiological explanations for their rationale, why these work, how little we need of each food group suggested for snacks, and why skipping them could set her up for overeating later, hence sabotaging her weight loss attempts. I told her: "I've been saying I should write a book on the hypoglycemic diet for years because I am convinced that **hypoglycemia** is a major reason why many fail to lose weight." She encouraged me to write such a book because most people don't know how to manage low blood sugar and that the solution is relatively simple to understand once it is explained.

She, like many of the patients and clients I have counseled over the past ten years, showed classic symptoms of **hypoglycemia** (low blood sugar). Most had never been diagnosed with the condition because they didn't happen to have an episode of low blood sugar at the time of routine blood tests. It is a condition that can occur one day but not the next. It is relatively simple to treat, with minor adjustments in eating patterns and food choice combinations.

The recommended changes can improve concentration, mood and **satiety** (the absence of hunger) necessary to stick to a low enough calorie-intake to promote weight loss.

When I ran into the doctor a few weeks later, I was happy to hear she was feeling better. She said that she no longer experienced the drop in energy and lack of concentration she once did in the afternoons, and was less hungry, therefore able to cut back on her portions at mealtimes after incorporating the suggested snacks into her daily routine.

I myself was diagnosed with **hypoglycemia** when graduating from university (bachelor degree in Business Administration) in 1987. I had not yet studied Nutrition, and I didn't understand the importance of regular meals, let alone snacks.

I had no food on hand one day because I was moving. I had bought a muffin and orange juice in the morning before going for an hour-long run. I had put off lunch because I was so busy doing errands before the move, and was getting ready to have my graduation picture taken. I kept thinking, "I'll eat something later...later". By suppertime, I was getting my picture taken when the last thing I recall saying before fainting was: "it's so hot" under the lights. Fortunately, the photographer caught my fall.

When I came to, I didn't know where I was, who she (the photographer) was, and I felt terrible. I recall thinking: "Wow, my body is so weak! I never thought a young (healthy) body could suddenly feel like it could die." The photographer sat me in a chair and said she was going to get me juice and crackers — great insight on her part! I passed out two more times in the chair before she could give me the snack.

The ambulance came and took me to the hospital where a blood test confirmed that I had low blood sugar. The doctor told me "you don't need to eat much, but eat often...once you have fainted, you most likely never will again, because you will recognize the uncomfortable feeling, and eat before your condition gets this bad." His tip was helpful but he did not explain which foods and in what combination would be most beneficial. Most doctors have limited training in Nutrition. This is not meant as criticism, but rather a statement of fact. We cannot expect doctors to be experts in all fields of health, hence the need for a multidisciplinary approach to healthcare. It would have been preferable to refer me to a Registered Dietitian for counseling. Would you seek legal advice from an architect? Would you ask your lawyer to design your house? Then why turn anywhere else than to a Registered Dietitian when seeking nutrition advice? I have given Nutrition classes to medical residents, and hope to have had a positive impact on the type of information they provide to their patients.

The eating plan suggested in this book is also safe for those who are uncertain whether or not they have **hypoglycemia.** If you just want to experiment with eating frequently throughout the day, try it and see if you feel more in control of your appetite, while having more energy and better concentration throughout your long busy days.

Unlike rigid diets, this one doesn't restrict you to a fixed set of menus. You get to choose the foods you would like to eat from the lists provided and make up your own meal plan. Think of it as a learning exercise. With repetition, you should have a good idea of portion sizes of the different food groups, and be able to eventually set the meal plan aside, only referring to it to refresh your memory.

1- WHAT IS HYPOGLYCEMIA (Low Blood Sugar)?

Hypoglycemia, or low blood sugar, occurs when blood levels of glucose (sugar) are too low to meet the energy demands of the body. Hypoglycemia is considered a condition, not a disease. It can be caused by individual hormonal irregularities or by an underlying disease. It can occur when levels drop below 3.8 mmol/L (SI unit) or 70 mg/dl (U.S. unit). Normal levels between meals should be 3.8 to 6.1 mmol/L (68 to 110 mg/dl). The exact level that is used to diagnose hypoglycemia varies somewhat depending on the source. The appearance of symptoms can occur at varying glucose levels for different individuals.[20]

According to the National Diabetes Clearing House of the U.S. National Institutes of Health,

> **Fasting hypoglycemia** is diagnosed from a blood sample that shows a blood glucose level of less than 50 mg/dl (2.8 mmol/L) after an overnight fast, between meals, or after exercise.... In **reactive hypoglycemia**, symptoms appear within 4 hours after you eat a meal.

> To diagnose **reactive hypoglycemia**, your doctor may

- Ask you about signs and symptoms;
- Test your blood glucose **while you are having symptoms** (The doctor will take a blood sample

from your arm and send it to a laboratory for analysis. A personal blood glucose monitor **cannot** be used to diagnose **reactive hypoglycemia**.);

- Check to see whether your symptoms ease after your blood glucose returns to 70 (3.8 mmol/L) or above (after eating or drinking).

A blood glucose level of less than 70 (3.8 mmol/L) at the time of symptoms and relief after eating will confirm the diagnosis.

The oral glucose tolerance test is no longer used to diagnose hypoglycemia; experts now know that the test can actually trigger hypoglycemic symptoms.[13]

As previously mentioned, it is difficult to detect the condition unless you have a blood test taken at a time when you happen to have an episode of low blood sugar. This can occur occasionally in some and more often in others. Because you would unlikely be able to coordinate a medical appointment at the time of symptoms, try monitoring your symptoms. Be aware that stress can trigger the same fight-or-flight hormones and hence lead to similar symptoms. Do you feel better when you eat more often and lousy when meals or snacks are delayed (**fasting hypoglycemia**)? Do you experience symptoms within 4 hours of a sugar-laden meal (**reactive hypoglycemia**, the less common form)?

If you have friends or family who test their blood sugar for diabetes, consider asking them to try their glucometer to test your blood sugar (blood glucose) at a time you have some of the symptoms listed below. As mentioned, a blood sample from your arm is more accurate but the glucometer may help to determine if you do experience hypoglycemia, particularly the less common type, **reactive hypoglycemia** (blood glucose below 3.8 mmol/L or 70 mg/dL) within four hours of eating. The most common form, **fasting hypoglycemia** is diagnosed at levels under 2.8 mmol/L (50 mg/dL). Although some glucometers may not be reliable at blood glucose levels below 3.3 mmol/L (60 mg/dL), the makers of the OneTouch® Ultra® System state that "the performance of OneTouch® Ultra® Test Strips has been evaluated both in laboratory and in clinical tests. It has been shown that the OneTouch® Ultra® compares well with a laboratory method. The OneTouch® Ultra® System has a measurement range of 1.1 to 33.3 mmol/L (20 to 600 mg/dL). (Reference: OneTouch® Ultra® Test Strip Insert AW06052707 Revision C)." If your reading is lower than normal or you experience symptoms, be sure to let your doctor know so that any serious underlying conditions may be ruled out.

Hypoglycemia can occur in some individuals for whom **insulin** and **glucagon** (hormones) production is not "fine tuned". They may not produce enough glucagon, insulin's counter regulating hormone, to tap into "sugar" reserves in their muscles and liver to transport "sugar" into the bloodstream in order to elevate blood glucose to a normal level. Other individuals may produce too much insulin after a meal or may be more sensitive to the affect of insulin (**reactive hypoglycemia**), hence transporting too much **glucose** from the blood to cells, leaving blood levels below normal range. The first condition can occur when meals are more than five hours apart or snacks are omitted (**fasting hypoglycemia**). The latter condition occurs 1½ to 4 hours after a meal (often rich in concentrated sweets), and is called **reactive hypoglycemia.**

CARBOHYDRATES EATEN ARE
BROKEN DOWN TO SUGAR
(GLUCOSE) IN THE DIGESTIVE
TRACT AND ABSORBED INTO
THE BLOOD STREAM

↓

ELEVATED BLOOD SUGAR
SIGNALS THE BODY TO
PRODUCE MORE INSULIN

↓

INSULIN TAKES SUGAR FROM
THE BLOOD STREAM AND
DIRECTS IT INTO THE CELL
TO BE USED AS FUEL

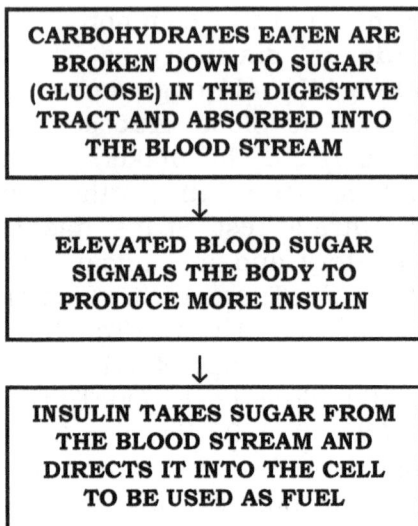

In **reactive hypoglycemia**, excessive insulin can be produced, causing too much "sugar" to be lead out of the blood stream into cells 1½ to 4 hours after eating. In f**asting hypoglycemia** (the most common form), an insufficient supply of absorbed "sugar" (digested carbohydrates) is available for the cells, including brain cells.

The resulting low blood sugar affects brain function (ex: may lead to reduced concentration, irritability). The brain cannot store adequate reserves of glucose; it depends on eaten sources or limited storage from muscle and liver reserves. The brain takes **glucose** ("sugar") and oxygen from the bloodstream to "feed itself". Glucose is the primary fuel source of the brain. The brain cannot store it, so it requires a steady supply in order to maintain normal functions. If blood levels of glucose drop, the body releases counter-regulatory hormones such as **glucagon**, epinepherine and norepinepherine. Glucagon has a function that is opposite to the function of insulin. Glucagon taps into "sugar" reserves (in the muscles and liver) and sends it into the bloodstream. Insulin, on the other hand, leads "sugar" from the bloodstream into the various cells of the body where it can be burned as fuel. Epinepherine and norepinepherine cause many of the fight-or-flight symptoms such as tremors, anxiety, palpitations, sweating and hunger. These can occur at blood sugar levels near 3.0 mmol/L (mid-50 mg/dL). Brain function is noticeably impaired at levels of 2.7 mmol/L (49 mg/dL) when signs like fatigue, confusion or strange behavior such as trouble speaking and lack of coordination may be experienced. It can be life-threatening if levels drop to around 1.9 mmol/L (mid-30 mg/dL). Blood sugar levels at which symptoms occur vary among individuals.

| HOURS FASTING OR INCREASED PHYSICAL ACTIVITY DEPLETE THE CARBOHYDRATE (SUGAR) FUEL SOURCE IN THE BLOOD STREAM |

OR

| EXCESS INSULIN PRODUCTION TAKES TOO MUCH BLOOD SUGAR OUT OF THE BLOOD STREAM |

↓

| LOW BLOOD SUGAR TRIGGERS COUNTER-REGULATORY HORMONE PRODUCTION (Ex: GLUCAGON) |

↓

| GLUCAGON TAPS INTO "SUGAR" RESERVES.(Ex: in liver) AND LEADS IT INTO THE BLOODSTREAM (ELEVATES BLOOD SUGAR). OTHER COUNTER-REGULATORY HORMONES CAUSE THE HYPOGLYCEMIC SYMPTOMS |

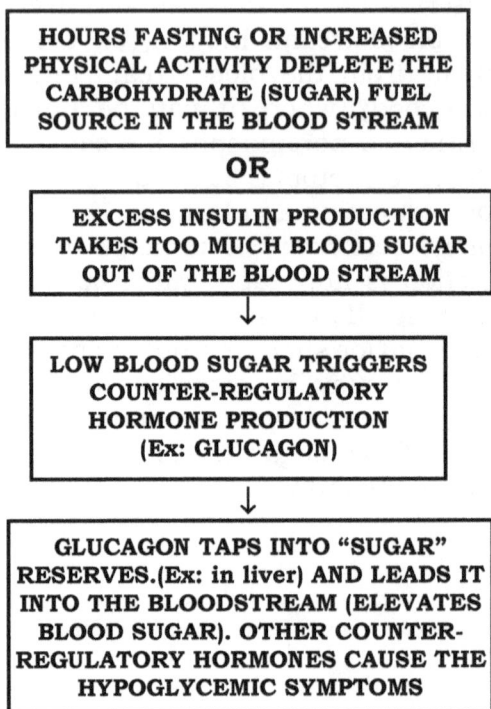

Could You Have This Condition (Hypoglycemia)?

Hypoglycemia can go undetected for years. You need not to have passed out to suspect low blood sugar. If you generally feel bad when meals are delayed, and then overeat to compensate, try this plan for a few weeks to see if it helps you feel better overall and more in control of your appetite.

Symptoms can include **hunger, irritability, trouble concentrating, anxiety, fatigue, headaches, weakness, sweating, dizziness, trembling, heart palpitations, blurred vision and loss of consciousness**. You may just experience any of the first four symptoms to a mild degree.

Increased caloric expenditure from running a long time and having gone too many hours without eating resulted in my fainting episode described in the Introduction. Much of the carbohydrate fuel in my bloodstream, muscles and liver had been depleted. My body was converting body tissue protein into the much-needed carbohydrates, but couldn't keep up with the demand. We faint when the brain is not nourished enough by oxygen or fuel (remember, glucose is the brain's indispensable fuel source). Falling down allows for greater blood flow to the brain in an attempt to nourish it.

If you do suspect hypoglycemia, please discuss the condition with your doctor to rule out any possible underlying diseases such as pancreatic or liver disease.

Although the advice in this book can help many significantly, I still suggest you consult a **Registered Dietitian** if you experience **hypoglycemia** or any other nutritionally related condition. A dietitian can evaluate your eating habits and ensure you are following the most appropriate meal plan for your condition as well as estimate your nutritional needs. The web site of the American Dietetic Association can assist you in finding a Registered Dietitian in your area (USA) at www.eatright.org. Canadian readers can locate one at www.dietitians.ca. Quebec readers can locate professional dietitians at www.opdq.org.

Could Low Blood Sugar Be Sabotaging Your Weight Loss Attempts?

Low blood sugar can lead to overeating — especially sweets. The hypoglycemic individual instinctively knows that **concentrated** sources of **simple sugars** will make them feel instantly better in the short run by raising blood sugar levels. Simple sugars are very quickly absorbed. White sugar, brown sugar, honey, syrup, molasses, jams, jelly, candy, soft drinks, ice cream, cookies, fruit punch and other sweets are some examples. The brain receives its preferred fuel source (glucose) rapidly. Its functions and your ability to concentrate improve. It is no longer a question of willpower to resist sweets, but rather one of sheer instinct to eat something sweet in order to relieve the discomfort. The downfall for individuals with **reactive hypoglycemia** is that they may produce too much **insulin** after a "sweet binge" and find themselves with low blood sugar once again. This can lead to a vicious cycle.

2- THE MEAL / SNACK MIX

Carbohydrates

The base of the human diet has consisted of **carbohydrates** for thousands of years. The Incas relied on corn; rice accounted for most of the caloric intake in China and India; wheat was eaten during the time of the Bible when feasts of sacrificed meat were served on special occasions, not everyday; legumes (dried beans, lentils, etc.) have been a staple in the Middle East and other regions for eons. Human metabolism has not suddenly evolved to function optimally on a diet consisting primarily of meat and/or fat even if a wave of fad diets might imply that.

Carbohydrates are made up of chains of **glucose** (the simplest form of carbohydrate). Carbohydrates are found in table sugar, honey syrup, jams, many desserts, candy, fruit, vegetables, potato, corn, rice, wheat and other grains. An introductory Biochemistry textbook tells us

> Since Acetyl-CoA is the end product of catabolism of fatty acids, we can see that mammals cannot exist with fats or acetate as the sole carbon source. The intermediates of carbohydrate metabolism would soon be depleted. **Carbohydrates are the principal energy and carbon source in animals**. Plants can carry out the conversion of acetyl-CoA to pyruvate and oxaloacetate, so they can exist without carbohydrates as carbon source.[4]

4- From *Biochemistry* 1st edition by Campbell. © 1991. Reprinted with permission of Brooks/Cole, a division of Thomson Learning: www.thomsonrights.com. Fax 800 730-2215.

Don't worry if the preceding paragraph is too technical. It is meant to illustrate that **carbohydrates** should be your main energy fuel (even for diabetics). Sugar has gotten an undeserved bad rap in recent years. It is not the evil villain it has been made out to be. Carbohydrates, whether simple or complex end up as **glucose** — sugar in its simplest form — once absorbed into the bloodstream. While knowing that, a balanced diet is not made up of an excess of any food source.

A **low-carbohydrate diet** is not an appropriate diet, especially for the **hypoglycemic** individual. It would deny them of the very nutrient they need most. Even **diabetics** should get most of their calories form carbohydrates.

Some of the **low-carbohydrate** fad diets discuss the action of **insulin** out of context. Their claims sound "scientific" and impressive, but in fact they do not consider the whole picture. For instance, some blame eating carbohydrates and subsequent rises in **insulin** levels as the leading cause for weight gain. Increased **insulin** will only result in gaining fat deposits if total calorie intake, whether from carbohydrates, protein or fat exceeds body needs. Otherwise, fat deposited after one meal will be burned off if there is a net deficit in total caloric intake for the day. An even balance of calories will result in weight maintenance; a deficit in caloric intake will result in weight loss, even if most calories come from carbohydrates.

Insulin not only directs glucose ("sugar") from the blood stream into cells but also fat and protein. Wanting to gain muscle? Don't go on a low-carbohydrate diet and lose the anabolic effect of insulin. Again, you will need a net increase in caloric intake to add muscle and weight. To associate carbohydrates alone with effects on insulin is not accurate.

High-calorie, low-fiber diets and inactivity are associated with obesity, not carbohydrate-rich diets including foods of high glycemic index. Many people believe that foods with a high glycemic index cause more fat storage by releasing more insulin. This is inaccurate because insulin release is both triggered by eating protein and magnified by the fat content of a meal. Excessive caloric intake ultimately leads to fat storage. High-carbohydrate, low to moderate fat diets are generally lower in calories (especially if they are high in fiber), and correlate with lower BMIs (**Body Mass Index**) than low-carbohydrate diets.

The **satiety index** and **energy density** lists can aid in choosing filling foods of lower calorie content in order to satisfy hunger while promoting weight loss by restricting calorie intake. Many dieters are unnecessarily avoiding carrots and potatoes. Please note that the terms energy and calorie may be used interchangeably.

One teaspoon of sugar provides only 16 calories. As previously mentioned, whether we eat starch, table sugar, honey or syrup, it all ends up as glucose ("sugar") when absorbed into the bloodstream. Now that you know this, try to avoid highly concentrated sweets such as soft drinks that contain approximately 10 teaspoons of sugar per can. This excessive intake of rapidly absorbed sugar could lead some individuals who tend to have **reactive hypoglycemic** episodes to produce excessive amounts of **insulin**, and a subsequent drop in blood sugar. Soft drinks are a leading cause of weight gain for many because it is easy to consume huge quantities of a liquid without feeling full. A 12-oz (355 mL) glass contains 150 calories. Some people are drinking 2 to 5 times this amount every day, hence 300 to 750 empty calories (of no nutritional value) per day. One need only cut 300 to 500 calories per day to promote weight loss. I once met a patient who told me she lost 30 pounds (13.6 kg) by simply cutting out the soft drinks from her diet. A simple look at the math explains this. I counseled another lady who was convinced that the teaspoon of sugar (16 calories) she added to her coffee every morning was making her fat. After analyzing her three-day food journal, it was clear that the 10-ounce steak (750 calories) was the source of most of her excess calories.

Those who experience **reactive hypoglycemia**, the less common form (occurs within 4 hours of eating), would do best to avoid **concentrated sweets** in order to avoid an excessive consumption of carbohydrates, followed by an excessive production of insulin that further drives blood sugar levels below normal range. This does not mean they may never be able to eat a small piece of cake or pie again. The once "forbidden foods" are even permitted in controlled amounts on most diabetic diets nowadays. Again, all carbohydrates, with the exception of fiber (it is not absorbed), end up as glucose when they are absorbed into the bloodstream. The issue with **concentrated sweets** is that in **reactive hypoglycemic** individuals, they can easily yield large quantities of rapidly absorbed glucose, causing a sudden rise in blood sugar and an overproduction of **insulin** to compensate. They may still tolerate small amounts taken in a combined protein, fat and fiber meal that would slow the carbohydrate absorption. Just avoid the **concentrated sweets** altogether in the beginning and monitor how you feel. You may be able to reintroduce small amounts later. The individual who suffers from **fasting hypoglycemia**, the more common form, may tolerate concentrated sweets without side effects. They should limit themselves to small quantities however, to avoid an excessive calorie intake if they are trying to lose weight.

Other examples of **concentrated sweets** (can be absorbed in less than 5 minutes) are

sugar	sweet pastries	ice cream
chocolate milk	brown sugar	gelatin dessert
puddings	honey	cakes
sherbet	molasses	fudge
jam	pies	jelly
icing	doughnuts	marmalade
chocolate bars	candy	syrups
sweetened beverages	cereal	regular chewing gum

Fruit, milk and vegetable sources of carbohydrate are also rapidly absorbed, but not as quickly as those in the list above. They take about 5 minutes to be absorbed. Because vegetables are relatively low in carbohydrates compared to fruit, milk and grain products or other starches, we must not rely on them as snacks to significantly raise blood sugar. Fruit, starch or milk choices are preferable.

Starches, such as bread, cereal, rice, pasta, potato and corn can take 20 minutes to digest, so if you have the "shakes", choose a small portion of a more rapidly absorbed source of carbohydrates such as a tablespoon (15 mL) of sugar or honey, or 4 ounces of orange juice. You should start to feel better within minutes if your blood sugar was low. Then follow with a **starch** plus a **protein choice** to sustain you. Remember, the use of concentrated sweets is to correct hypoglycemic episodes. The starch or fruit, with meat or fat is to prevent them.

Be careful not to choose low-carbohydrate bars containing primarily **sugar alcohols** for snacks as a means to prevent drops in blood sugar. **Xylitol, maltitol, sorbitol**, etc. are less absorbed than sugar or starch and won't result in the rise in blood sugar that you need. **Polydextrose** is a sugar substitute that is not absorbed through digestion therefore it won't raise blood sugar. A friend of mine who experienced **hypoglycemia** frequently in part because she was convinced that carbohydrates were "bad" and should be avoided, relied on a low-carbohydrate bar (containing primarily polydextrose as the sugar substitute) to prevent low blood sugar midday only to find herself trembling after eating one. This could have been dangerous, especially if she had been driving.

To Carb or Not To Carb?

A low-carbohydrate, high-protein diet is not recommended for weight-loss. It can be lacking in vital nutrients from fruits and vegetables, and high in fat, therefore high in calories. Eating too much **saturated fat** (fat that is solid at room temperature) can lead to heart disease, and an excessive protein intake may strain the kidneys and liver.

When a diet is low in carbohydrates (sugars, whether starches or simple sugars):

- the body's stores of carbohydrates that are in the form of **glycogen** are quickly depleted. Because each molecule of glycogen is bound to almost 3 molecules of water, much needed body water is often lost with this use of glycogen, giving the dieter a false sense of fat loss when the scale reading drops. This can lead to dehydration, which is particularly risky if one is exercising.

- because the brain and red blood cells are glucose (carbohydrate) dependent (they are unable to rely solely on fat stores in the body for energy), the body resorts to breaking down its tissues such as muscle and dietary protein to convert this protein to the much-needed carbohydrates. This results in a **loss of lean body mass** (noticed when you hop on the scale) — something you don't want to lose, especially if you want to lose body fat. The loss of lean body tissue results in a **decrease in metabolic rate** (the number of calories the body burns each day), setting the dieter up for failure in the long run and now gaining weight on the same number of calories they once maintained, or even lost weight on.

- when the body primarily relies on fat for energy, a build-up of a by-product called **ketones** results in **ketosis** that leads to muscle breakdown, nausea, dehydration, light-headedness, irritability, bad breath, headaches, kidney problems, and may cause fetal abnormality or death. It can be fatal for diabetics.

A diet rich in carbohydrates with moderate amounts of protein and fat is recommended for weight loss.

Dietitians have recommended low to moderate fat intake for decades. Some people misunderstood this and assumed that eating "almost no fat" would be better. Extremely low-fat diets left many feeling hungry in between meals because fat as well as protein slow stomach emptying, hence increase satiety. Remember, 20 to 35% of calories from fat can allow most adults a teaspoon or two of added fat with each meal.

For those who suffer from **hypoglycemia** (lower than normal blood sugar), they often feel hunger and an almost instinctive urge to eat carbohydrates. Eating 3 meals and 3 snacks containing mainly carbohydrates and modest amounts of protein and fat helps to control appetite by maintaining blood sugar within a normal range, hence improving satiety between meals.

Keep in mind that cutting calories below the amount "burned" each day, will result in weight loss, whether the calories cut from the diet are primarily from carbohydrate, protein or fat (the only 3 sources of calories besides alcohol).

The healthiest way to lose weight is still by following Canada's Food Guide or the United States Department of Agriculture Food Guide Pyramid (www.mypyramide.gov/). The latter may help you calculate individual food portions to promote weight loss on a balanced diet by getting most of your calories from carbohydrates and cutting back on portions and high-fat foods (they have more than twice the amount of calories per weight compared to carbohydrates and protein). Fill up on high volume foods of **low caloric density** (ex: high fiber fruit, veggies and whole grains, but limit fruit juice intake to 4-oz servings). Even if you "over-indulge", it is preferable to have those extra calories come from carbohydrates because the body will burn some of those calories trying to convert them into fat, whereas dietary fat can be deposited in fat stores without a significant energy expenditure.

Our bodies were designed to function with a diet providing **most of its calories from carbohydrates**, so please don't be mislead by the latest low-carbohydrate craze. Any diet that suggests avoiding the base of the Food Guide Pyramid (breads, cereals, rice, pastas, fruit and vegetables) is likely to set the dieter up for long-term failure and increase their health risks [ex: cancers (fruit and vegetables are rich in phytochemicals, antioxidants and fiber) and coronary artery diseases].

For individualized help in designing a healthy meal plan to meet your needs consult a **Registered Dietitian (RD)** or a **Professional Dietitian, PDt,** in Quebec.

Protein

High **protein** foods include meat, fish, poultry, eggs, dairy products (milk, yogurt and cheeses), **legumes** (dried beans, lentils, chickpeas, etc.) and seed and nuts.

Digestion of **protein** begins in the stomach, hence, proteins slow stomach emptying and increases **satiety** ("the feeling of fullness or satisfaction after a meal"[15]). You need not eat large quantities of protein to reduce hunger.

Most people don't need more than six ounces of meat or equivalent alternatives per day. (See Chapter 6 - Building Your Personalized Meal Plan to estimate your needs). The size of a deck of cards of cooked meat or poultry or the size of a checkbook of fish are all about 3 oz. Having 1 oz with snacks is usually sufficient (ex: 1 oz of low-fat cheese is roughly the size of a large dice or one-inch or 2.5 cm cube).

Fat

Oil, margarine, butter, mayonnaise and salad dressings are considered as added fats (fats we add to our meal). Fat is already in much of the food we eat for example, meats, fish, eggs, cheese, milk (except skim), cheeses, avocado, olives, French fries, crackers, pie crusts, cookies, etc.

Although fat digestion begins in the mouth, 20 to 30% of its digestion occurs in the stomach where enzymes are most activated due to the acidic environment. When fat enters the small intestine, a hormone named enterogastrone is believed to slow stomach emptying by decreasing motility and stomach secretions.

We don't need to consume large amounts of fat either. Essential fatty acids must come from the diet. A minimum of 3% of calories from omega-6 fatty acids and 0.5% from omega-3 are suggested (1% if no **EPA** and **DHA** from fish are consumed). One can easily consume sufficient omega-6 fatty acids on even very low-fat diet, such as 10 to 15% fat. It takes more planning to get enough omega-3 fatty acids to improve the ratio of omega-6 to omega-3. A tablespoon (15 mL) of soybean oil or walnut oil per day would meet the requirements of a 2000-calorie diet for example. If you like fish, try to have 3 or more servings of the "fatty" (cold water) varieties such as salmon, tuna and trout per week. Adding 3 to 6 teaspoons (15 to 30 mL) of added fat per day is sufficient to meet the nutritional needs of most people. A teaspoon of mayonnaise added to your sandwich, or 1 to 2 teaspoons of oil to your salad is all that is needed at mealtime to increase **satiety**.

The reason I repeatedly suggest low-fat versions of snack foods is because fat has 9 calories per gram as opposed to 4 per gram of carbohydrate or protein. I suggest high volume, low calorie choices to fill you up, and to promote weight loss. Since fat is the most concentrated source of calories, choosing low fat foods can allow for high volumes with less calories. This gives you more food for your buck, so to speak. This does not mean one should avoid a serving or two of nutritious oils per meal; they are associated with many health benefits. The total calories consumed minus the total calories burned in a day, is what ultimately counts when it comes to weight loss. The goal is to keep total caloric intake low enough to promote a loss of excess weight while increasing **satiety**.

When an item is a rich source of **saturated fat** such as cheese, I do recommend a low-fat version. Consider starting with 15% **M.F.** and gradually "weaning" your way down to 8% **M.F.** (or less) cheeses. It is as easy as converting from whole milk, to 2%, to 1%. With time, one can learn to enjoy these choices, and even find that the higher fat versions they once enjoyed, become unappealing. Many who have progressed to 1% or skim milk no longer tolerate whole milk because they now find the texture too thick, even though they once enjoyed whole milk and fussed at the suggestion of switching to a low-fat version.

Alcohol

Alcohol is the only other dietary source of calories besides **carbohydrate**, **protein** and **fat**. It is relatively high in calories with 7 calories per gram *versus* 4 calories per gram of **carbohydrate** and **protein**, and 9 calories per gram of **fat.**

Alcohol does not raise blood sugar unless it's a "sweet drink" or beer. It could cause blood sugar to drop (**hypoglycemia**) however by affecting the body's conversion of protein and fat into **glucose** (carbohydrate) by a process called **gluconeogenesis that** occurs in the liver.

It is a good idea to avoid alcohol if you experience **hypoglycemia.** If you choose to drink, do so occasionally, and in moderation (1 to 2 drinks). Have it with a meal or snack containing **carbohydrates** (Ex: pasta or Melba Toast), and do not drive. Alcoholic beverages can lead to a significant intake of empty calories. Drinking 2 martinis (312 calories) for example, could sabotage your aim to reduce your intake by 300 to 500 calories/day to lose weight.

CALORIC CONTENT OF VARIOUS ALCOHOLIC BEVERAGES

12 oz (355 mL) beer	153 calories
1.5 oz (44 mL) gin, rum, vodka or whiskey (80 proof)	97 calories
3.5 oz (104 mL) table wine	87 calories

THE MEAL / SNACK MIX

Meals

Try to use most of the food groups with each meal. For example,

BREAKFAST
Grain Product	2 whole-wheat toast
Fruit	1 orange
Dairy	1 cup (240 mL) 1% milk
Meat or Alternative	1 egg
Fat	2 tsp (10 mL) peanut butter

LUNCH
Grain Product	sandwich on rye bread
Fruit	15 grapes
Vegetable	1 cup (240) cucumber
Dairy	¾ cup (180 mL) yogurt
Meat or Alternative	2 oz (60 g) turkey
Fat	1 tsp (5 mL) mayo

DINNER
Grain Product	1 cup brown rice
Fruit	½ banana
Vegetable	2 cups (500 mL) salad
Dairy	1 cup (240 mL) 1% milk
Meat or Alternative	3 oz (90 g) salmon
Fat	1 Tbs (15 mL) olive oil dressing

Snacks

Choose snacks with a **carbohydrate-choice (starch or grain product, fruit or dairy)** and combine with either a **protein or fat-choic**e to slow digestion, hence the absorption of the carbohydrates ingested. For example,

- 4 whole grain Melba Toast with 2 tsp (10 mL) peanut-butter
- 1 apple with 1 oz (30 g) of low-fat cheese

Select any item from the **starch (grain)**, **fruit** or **dairy** group and **combine** it with a selection from the **protein** or **fat (or dairy)** group. Mix and match snack choices from the following pages.

AM SNACK
CARB-CHOICE
Grain Product   4 whole grain Melba toast
OR   OR
Fruit   1 apple
OR   OR
Dairy   ¾ cup (180 mL) yogurt
                           (low-fat, sugar-free)

WITH

PROTEIN-CHOICE
Dairy   1 cup (240 mL) 1% milk
OR   OR
Meat or Alternative   1 oz cheese
OR   OR

FAT-CHOICE
Fat   2 tsp peanut butter

AFTERNOON SNACK

CARB-CHOICE

Grain Product	2 rice cakes
OR	OR
Fruit	1 peach
OR	OR
Dairy	¾ cup (180 mL) yogurt (low-fat, sugar-free)

WITH

PROTEIN-CHOICE

Dairy	¾ cup (180 mL) yogurt (low-fat, sugar-free)
OR	OR
Meat or Alternative	1 oz (30 g) ham
OR	OR

FAT-CHOICE

Fat	6 almonds

EVENING SNACK

CARB-CHOICE

Grain Product	¾ cup of cereal
OR	OR
Fruit	1¼ cup (300 mL) berries
OR	OR
Dairy	1 cup (240 mL) 1% milk

WITH

PROTEIN-CHOICE

Dairy	1 cup (240 mL) 1% milk
OR	OR
Meat or Alternative	1 boiled egg
OR	OR

FAT-CHOICE

Fat	8 large olives

Some practical snack choices are those containing both protein and fat in the same food item such as low-fat cheese or natural (**non-hydrogenated**) peanut butter, which also contains fiber, another high-satiety ingredient.

Be sure not to skip your evening snack if you are waking up at night feeling hungry.

If your blood cholesterol levels are normal and you are not considered at high risk for heart disease (check with your doctor) it is considered safe to eat up to one egg (yolk) per day. If your cholesterol level is high however, limit to two egg yolks per week.

Be prepared! Always have snacks on hand. Keep Melba Toast and nuts in your desk, fruit and cheese in your lunch bag, cereal or nutritious bars in your glove compartment or purse. PRIA™ is an example of a low-calorie bar (110 calories in those sold in the USA and 170 calories in those sold in Canada) containing a mix of carbohydrate, a little protein and fat. Others include LUNA®, the Whole Nutrition Bar for Women™ (180 calories) as well as EQUIBARS™ by BIOETIK® that are made of organic ingredients such as brown rice syrup, almond butter, dried fruit and hemp seeds. Their flavors include: cranberry bar (120 calories), fig, peanut butter & carob, apricot bars (140 calories), blueberry bar (150 calories), almond bar (170 calories) or almond & carob bar (180 calories). EQUIBARS™ are only available in Canada at this time.

Try cooking large batches of meals that can be frozen and quickly reheated on days you get home late. This will help you to avoid delaying meals any further. Order groceries to be delivered if you don't have time to shop.

3- HOW TO MANAGE HYPOGLYCEMIA

Timing Meals and Snacks

Eating meals and snacks at regular intervals has to become a priority for the individual with **hypoglycemia.** For them, this is much like taking medication at prescribed times. Meals and snacks should be eaten approximately **3 hours apart** if having 3 meals and 3 snacks per day. Otherwise, try to have meals no more than 5 hours apart if any of the snacks are omitted.

Ex:			Shift worker
		OR	**OR**
Breakfast	7:00 AM	6:30	5:00 PM
Snack	10:00 AM	9:30 AM	8:00 PM
Lunch	1:00PM	NOON	11:00 PM
Snack	4:00 PM	3:00 PM	2:00 AM
Dinner	7:00 PM	5:30 PM	5:00 AM
Snack	10:00 PM	8:00 PM	8:00 AM

Don't worry. Calories eaten at night are not more fattening than those eaten midday. Remember, the total calorie intake of the day is what counts. As long as you do not exceed your calorie needs for the day, your body will later tap into fat deposited from calories eaten in the evening.

Be sure not to skip breakfast. Stores of carbohydrate in the liver called **glycogen** may be depleted from having fasted overnight. If you enjoy a morning workout, it is even more important to replenish your carbohydrate stores before exercising. Otherwise, you would be trying to "run on empty" and could either experience low blood sugar or break down muscle to convert to carbohydrate for fuel. Remember, losing muscle results in a lower metabolic rate hence, fewer calories are burned.

Some may find they don't feel the need for a morning snack but experience low energy and concentration levels mid-afternoon, around 3 PM, and are hungry in the evening. I suggest starting with 3 meals and 3 snacks for a week or so to see how you feel. You may later eliminate a snack or 2 if you feel they are not always needed. It is still a good idea to keep some snacks readily available in the event you suddenly feel the symptoms described earlier (hunger, inability to concentrate, irritability, shakiness, weakness, etc.). Again, if you are not sure whether or not you have **hypoglycemia**, try this pattern of eating for two weeks and note how you feel.

If after your two-week trial of 3 meals and 3 snacks per day, you only feel the need for an afternoon snack, try to have breakfast and lunch within a five-hour interval, and a three-hour interval between lunch, your PM snack and dinner.
Ex: Breakfast at 7AM, lunch at noon, a snack at 3 PM and dinner at 6 PM. If your boss or colleagues frown at the idea of your needing to take a short break and snack mid-morning and mid-afternoon, assure them that it will only make you more productive.

What to Eat

"All foods can fit" into your meal plan, but if you want to lose weight, aim for **high volume/low calorie choices** most often. When indulging in a piece of high calorie cake or pie for example, have a small piece and avoid doing so on an empty stomach. This will make it easier to keep portions small.

Consider keeping "trigger foods" out of the house for the first few months. These are foods that you do not feel you can stop at just one portion. When craving chips for example, go out and buy one individual serving size of baked chips. If you crave ice cream, go to a local parlor and buy a low-fat ice cream cone and savor it. Avoid doing so on an empty stomach in order to prevent yourself from overindulging. Eventually you should be tuned into your symptoms of low blood sugar and able to prevent their occurrence more often. Then your "trigger food" should become just another food in your cupboard that you enjoy once in a while in moderation because you are able to avoid periods of low blood sugar, have less frequent cravings and fewer periods of intense hunger.

Diet for Hypoglycemia

It is important to not skip meals and to eat at even intervals (ex: 5 to 6 hour intervals between meals). Snacks containing complex carbohydrates along with some protein and fat (protein and fat slow stomach emptying), scheduled in between meals are recommended to prevent drops in blood sugar.

Concentrated sweets such as **table sugar, brown sugar, honey, molasses, regular soft drinks, syrups, regular jams, marshmallow, candy and chocolate bars** and products containing them in high concentration should be avoided to prevent **reactive hypoglycemia**, which leads to an increase in **insulin** release, which in turn could cause a further drop in blood sugar. It is a good idea to **avoid large quantities** of these foods for anyone trying to cut calories in order to lose weight.

FOOD GROUP	SUGGESTED FOODS
GRAIN PRODUCTS	Whole-grain or enriched breads, cereals, rice, pastas and barley
VEGETABLES	All fresh, frozen, canned or vegetable juices
FRUITS	All fresh, frozen or canned (packed in their own juice, no sugar added) Fruit juice (no sugar added) Dried fruit in moderation
MILK AND YOGURT	Milk, unsweetened yogurt
MEATS, FISH, POULTRY, CHEESE DRIED BEANS, NUTS AND EGGS	Meat, fish, poultry, cheese, dried beans or lentils, nuts and seeds Eggs

FOOD GROUP	FOODS TO AVOID WITH REACTIVE HYPOGLYCEMIA OR TO REDUCE CALORIES
GRAIN PRODUCTS	Sweet pastries (ex: cakes, cookies, doughnuts), highly sweetened cereals, rice pudding
VEGETABLES	Candied yams, brown sugar or syrup coated vegetables
FRUITS	Candied fruit, fruit packed in sweetened syrup
MILK AND YOGURT	Sweetened yogurt, milkshakes, chocolate milk, ice cream, sherbet
MEATS, FISH, POULTRY, CHEESE DRIED BEANS, NUTS AND EGGS	Baked beans with molasses, meat, fish or poultry topped with sweet sauce, sweet dessert or candy

SAMPLE MENU TO MANAGE HYPOGLYCEMIA

BREAKFAST 7AM
Oatmeal (½ cup, 125 mL)
Skim milk (8 oz, 240 mL)
Slice whole wheat toast
Egg
½ banana

AM SNACK   10 AM
2 rice cakes
Peanut butter (preferably non-hydrogenated)
(2 tsp, 10 mL)

LUNCH   NOON
Turkey (2 to 3 oz, 60 to 90 g) sandwich
        on whole wheat bread
Mayonnaise (1 tsp, 5 mL)
Carrots and cucumber
Orange
Unsweetened yogurt (maximum 2% M.F.)
        (¾ cup, 180 mL)

PM SNACK   3 PM
6 soda crackers
Cheese (maximum 15% M.F.) (1 oz, 30 g)

SUPPER   5 PM
Fish (3 oz, 90 g)
Brown rice (1 cup, 240 mL)
Mixed vegetables
Fruit salad (½ cup, 125 mL)

EVENING SNACK   8 PM
Bowl of whole grain cereal (unsweetened)
        (¾ cup, 180 mL)
Skim milk (½ cup, 125 mL)

Managing hypoglycemia involves **PREVENTING EPISODES OF LOW BLOOD SUGAR BEFORE THEY OCCUR.**

4- HIGH SATIETY FOODS

How to curb appetite

High satiety foods are shown to decrease appetite for extended periods of time.

Why is fiber important?

Fiber adds bulk to food, but it is indigestible, therefore does not provide calories. Actually, the number of grams of fiber may be subtracted from the total grams of carbohydrates in a food serving to determine the amount of carbohydrate absorbed. Once ingested, fiber absorbs water in the digestive tract adding to its weight that in turn makes us feel fuller. It helps avoid constipation by increasing stool volume.

When hungry, choose foods with higher indexes (percentage) from the **high satiety list** (pages 43 to 44). Many are high in fiber and/or protein, the two factors that slow stomach emptying. Try to choose foods that also have a **low energy density** (calories per pound of food) to promote weight loss (pages 45 to 46). **Legumes (dried bean, lentils, chickpeas, split peas**, etc), are good examples of high satiety foods. They are also low in both fat and calories, making them a great diet choice. One evening, I was at a restaurant with a group of at least 12 people. Most of us ordered lentil soup with plain bread to start. By the time the main course arrived, we were all too full to eat anything else whether young, old, male, female, slim or heavy.

If you avoid **legumes** because of the flatulence (gas) they may cause, build up your tolerance gradually and try not to eat them at multiple meals in a row. Beano™ can relieve this symptom. It contains an enzyme that allows you to break down and absorb the fiber that causes flatulence as a result of bacterial **fermentation** of the indigestible carbohydrates. I suggest that you do not use an enzyme to break down fiber often. Much of the benefits of fiber come from the very fact that it is indigestible: fewer calories are absorbed. **Soluble fiber** lowers cholesterol and slows carbohydrate absorption and hence helps to prevent sudden rises in blood sugar in diabetics. It also increases **satiety**. Perhaps Beano™ could be saved for times when you have social engagements.

Another key to increasing **satiety** is to eat foods that are "heavy" in the stomach but low in calories to promote weight loss. We tend to eat roughly the same weight of food each day. Aim for foods of high volume but low to moderate in calories.

Opposite examples of high satiety foods are soft drinks and ice cream. As previously mentioned, liquids are not very filling (with the exception of a fruit smoothie because it is heavy, contains fiber from the fruit and protein from the milk or yogurt). Ice cream is in a liquid form by the time we swallow it, so it is easy to consume a lot of it. Most people can easily drink 1½ to 2 liters (quarts) of liquid per day. Some are drinking this volume of soft drinks or a few cups of juice every day. Juice provides 60 calories per ½ cup (120 mL). If this portion feels like a tease, eat a small orange instead for the same amount of calories. Fresh fruit is more filling due to its fiber content. Try to get most of your fruit servings from fresh fruit and most of your hydration from water if you are trying to shed pounds. Regular vanilla ice cream is made of 10% fat. A rich variety may have 16% fat. They provide approximately 133 to 178 calories per 125 mL (or ½ cup) respectively. Some richer flavored varieties provide 270 calories per serving and macadamia nut ice cream may have as much as 360 calories per ½ cup. Servings often exceed ½ cup, so it is easy to understand why they can lead to weight gain. When choosing such foods, try the lower calorie versions. There are many great tasting low fat/low-sugar ice creams on the market. If you can't kick the soft drink habit, have a diet soft drink or consider switching to a sugar-free beverage such as Crystal Light™.

A croissant scores low on the satiety index list and high on the energy density list because it is light, made of white flour (no fiber) with butter between each layer of pastry. It isn't very filling, yet it's rich in calories (due primarily to the high butter content).

Low Energy Density Foods

These are foods of relatively low caloric content per weight. To curb appetite and promote weight loss, eat a high volume of food providing fewer calories. Does this mean you will never over-indulge again? Not likely, but the incidences should be less frequent and you should become aware of what might have led to it (for example, a skipped meal or snack leading to a drop in blood sugar, or a meal with little or no carbohydrates), and therefore be better able to prevent it from reoccurring frequently. Other factors such as Premenstrual Syndrome (PMS) may increase appetite and cravings. I say: "PMS is real!" Check your calendar to see if indulgences tend to occur seven to ten days prior to menstruation. (See Chapter 10- *Body Chemistry & Appetite*).

Satiety Index (SI) and Energy Density (ED)

Some suggested choices of **foods with high satiety indexes** are underlined in the list on the following pages. Foods such as popcorn, wheat bran, oatmeal, rice (white and brown), potatoes, whole grain bread and pasta, lentils, eggs, beans, beef, cod, grapes, apples and oranges were found to keep people satisfied longer (had a higher **satiety index**) than foods such as croissant, cake, doughnuts and candy bars. Yogurt, oatmeal, whole wheat pasta, brown rice, baked potato, lentils, baked beans, cod fish, banana, grapes, apples and oranges have a relatively low calorie level, as indicated on the **energy density list**.

SATIETY INDEX (average):
Choose foods with high satiety (%) when hungry
(All foods compare with white bread, 100%)

Bakery Products

Croissant	47%
Cake	65%
Doughnuts	68%
Cookies	120%
Crackers	127%

Snacks and Confectionary

MARS™ bar	70%
Peanuts	84%
Yogurt	88%
Chips	91%
Ice-cream	96%
Jellybeans	118%
Popcorn	154%

Breakfast Cereals with milk

Müeslix	100%
SUSTAIN™	112%
SPECIAL K™	116%
CORNFLAKES™	118%
HONEYSMACKS™	132%
ALL-BRAN™	151%
Porridge/Oatmeal	209%

Protein-Rich Foods

Lentils	133%
Cheese	146%
Eggs	150%
Baked beans	168%
Beef	176%
Ling fish (cod)	225%

Starch-Rich Foods

White bread	100%
French fries	116%
White pasta	119%
Brown Rice	132%
White rice	138%
Grain bread	154%
Wholemeal bread	157%
Brown pasta	188%
Potatoes	323%

Fruit

Bananas	118%
Grapes	162%
Apples	197%
Oranges	202%

Table adapted by permission from Macmillan Publishers Ltd: European Journal of Clinical Nutrition. S.H.A. Holt, J.C. Brand Miller, P. Petocz, and E. Farmakalidis: A Satiety Index of Common Foods. Table 4. 49: 9; 675-690 (1995).

ENERGY DENSITY:

Choose more often those foods with a low energy (caloric) density. Calories per pound (kcal/lb)

Food	kcal/lb
Bakery Products	
Cake, white	2006
Cookies	1956
Crackers	1967
Croissant	1771
Doughnuts	1760
Snacks and Confectionary	
Ice-cream chocolate	984
Jellybeans	1664
MARS™ bar	2116
Peanuts	2560
Popcorn	2384
Yogurt	278
Breakfast Cereals with Milk	
ALL-BRAN™	1120
CORNFLAKES™	1760
HONEYSMACKS™	1760
Müeslix	1689
Oatmeal	281
SUSTAIN™	1650
SPECIAL K™	1760
Starch-Rich Foods	
Brown rice	503
French fries	1415
Potato, baked	494
White pasta	639
Whole wheat bread	1056
Whole wheat pasta	564
White bread	1120
White rice	591

Protein-Rich Foods

Baked beans	648
Beef, round tip lean	817
Cheese, cheddar	1856
Cod fish	507
Eggs, hardboiled	700
Lentils	530

Fruit

Apples	266
Banana	418
Grapes	334
Oranges	211

Notice how **whole grain** breads, pasta and cereals score higher on the **satiety index** list. Even though white rice scored higher than brown, I still suggest opting for the brown rice because of its high fiber content and superior nutritional value. It is a better choice on the **energy density** list (lower in calories per weight *versus* white rice). Cake, croissant, doughnuts and candy bars score low in terms of **satiety index** but score high in **energy density**. These are not very filling but loaded with calories, therefore not the best choices.

It is possible to lose weight without feeling famished.

5- ESTIMATING CALORIC NEEDS

If you would rather not calculate your estimated caloric needs, use the charts below to estimate your calorie level based on gender, age and activity level.

Caloric Needs for Females by Activity Level and Age

AGE	ACTIVITY LEVELS		
	Sedentary*	Moderately active*	Active*
19 to 20	2000	2200	2400
21 to 25	2000	2200	2400
26 to 30	1800	2000	2400
31 to 35	1800	2000	2200
36 to 40	1800	2000	2200
41 to 45	1800	2000	2200
46 to 50	1800	2000	2200
51 to 55	1600	1800	2200
56 to 60	1600	1800	2200
61 to 65	1600	1800	2000
66 to 70	1600	1800	2000
71 to 75	1600	1800	2000
76 and older	1600	1800	2000

Caloric Needs for Males by Activity Level and Age

AGE	ACTIVITY LEVELS		
	Sedentary*	Moderately active*	Active*
19 to 20	2600	2800	3000
21 to 25	2400	2800	3000
26 to 30	2400	2600	3000
31 to 35	2400	2600	3000
36 to 40	2400	2600	2800
41 to 45	2200	2600	2800
46 to 50	2200	2400	2800
51 to 55	2200	2400	2800
56 to 60	2200	2400	2600
61 to 65	2000	2400	2600
66 to 70	2000	2200	2600
71 to 75	2000	2200	2600
76 and older	2000	2200	2400

"*Calorie levels are based on the Estimated Energy Requirements (EER and activity levels from the Institute of Medicine Dietary Reference Intakes Macronutrients Report, 2002.

SEDENTARY = less than 30 minutes per day of moderate physical activity in addition to daily activities.

MODERATELY ACTIVE = at least 30 minutes up to 60 minutes per day of moderate physical activity in addition to daily activities.

ACTIVE = 60 or more minutes per day of moderate physical activity in addition to daily activities."

Adapted from "MyPyramid Food Intake Pattern Calorie Levels" source: United States Department of Agriculture Center for Nutrition Policy and Promotion. April 2005 CNPP-XX

You may also go to www.mypyramid.gov
to get a quick estimate of your caloric needs and

recommended portions based on your age, gender and activity level.

Keep in mind that we are initially estimating the number of calories to maintain your current weight. For weight loss, subtract 300 to 500 calories. For those wishing to increase weight, add 300 to 500 calories to determine your meal plan calorie level. A reduction of 3500 calories results in one pound of weight lost. Subtracting 500 calories per day would theoretically result in one pound lost per week. However, other factors such as varied activity level day-to-day, net decrease from habitual consumption all enter into the weight loss equation. This is why a 300 calorie-a-day reduction from estimated needs is often sufficient to lose weight.

You will start with an estimated calorie amount to promote weight loss. Notice that the formulas are only estimates and yield varying results. So it may be necessary to adjust your meal plan level (calorie level) based on your weight loss results. If you are losing less or more than 1 to 2 pounds per week, reduce or increase by another 300 calories, accordingly. Rapid weight loss can be the result of muscle loss. This should be avoided as much as possible because muscle is metabolically active (burns calories).

It is a good idea to incorporate weight-bearing exercise such as free weights, weight machines, Pilates or other types according to your capacities and the permission of your physician. You need to prevent muscle loss and to prevent reaching a plateau before attaining your weight loss goal.

For those who would like to calculate their estimated caloric needs, the following equations may be used.

Before calculating your caloric needs, begin by determining your desirable body weight and **Body Mass Index (BMI).**

Body Mass Index

The Body Mass Index is the result when you divide your weight in kilograms (kg) by your height in meters squared.

If you would rather skip the equation, simply refer to the following tables. Find your height along the left-hand column of the table, and look across the row until you find the number that is closest to your weight. The number at the top of the corresponding column identifies your BMI.

The BMI correlates with disease risks and can be used to classify obesity. It is most appropriate for 20- to 65-year-olds, excluding athletes, pregnant women or those who are breastfeeding.

A person measuring 5'5" tall and weighing 170 pounds would look up their height on the following chart in the far left column and find the weight closest to his in that corresponding row, which is 168 pounds. The corresponding column is that of a BMI of 28.

A BMI of 18.5 to 24.9 is considered desirable. Even if you do not reach this zone but manage to reduce your BMI from 30 to 27 for example, and maintain this weight, you can significantly reduce health risks.

Body Mass Index (BMI)

Height	18	19	20	21	22	23	24	25	26	27
				Body weight (pounds)						
4'11"	89	94	99	104	109	114	119	124	128	133
5'0"	92	97	102	107	112	118	123	128	133	138
5'1"	95	100	106	111	116	122	127	132	137	143
5'2"	98	104	109	115	120	126	131	136	142	147
5'3"	102	107	113	118	124	130	135	141	146	152
5'4"	105	110	116	122	128	134	140	145	151	157
5'5"	108	114	120	126	132	138	144	150	156	162
5'6"	112	118	124	130	136	142	148	155	161	167
5'7"	115	121	127	134	140	146	153	159	166	172
5'8"	118	125	131	138	144	151	158	164	171	177
5'9"	122	128	135	142	149	155	162	169	176	182
5'10"	126	132	139	146	153	160	167	174	181	188
5'11"	129	136	143	150	157	165	172	179	186	193
6'0"	132	140	147	154	162	169	177	184	191	199
6'1"	136	144	151	159	166	174	182	189	197	204
6'2"	141	148	155	163	171	179	186	194	202	210
6'3"	144	152	160	168	176	184	192	200	208	216

Continued

Body Mass Index (BMI)

	28	29	30	31	32	33	34	35	36	37
Height				**Body weight (pounds)**						
4'11"	138	143	148	153	158	163	168	173	178	183
5'0"	143	148	153	158	163	168	174	179	184	189
5'1"	148	153	158	164	169	174	180	185	190	195
5'2"	153	158	164	169	175	180	186	191	196	202
5'3"	158	163	169	175	180	186	191	197	203	208
5'4"	163	169	174	180	186	192	197	204	209	215
5'5"	168	174	180	186	192	198	204	210	216	222
5'6"	173	179	186	192	198	204	210	216	223	229
5'7"	178	185	191	198	204	211	217	223	230	236
5'8"	184	190	197	203	210	216	223	230	236	243
5'9"	189	196	203	209	216	223	230	236	243	250
5'10"	195	202	209	216	222	229	236	243	250	257
5'11"	200	208	215	222	229	236	243	250	257	265
6'0"	206	213	221	228	235	242	250	258	265	272
6'1"	212	219	227	235	242	250	257	265	272	280
6'2"	218	225	233	241	249	256	264	272	280	287
6'3"	224	232	240	248	256	264	272	279	287	295

BMI = weight in kg / height in m2

**Under-
weight**
(< 18.5)

Healthy Weight
(18.5 to 24.9)

Overweight
(25 to 29.9)

Obese
(> = 30)

A BMI of 27 is acceptable for persons aged 65 years or more

Moderate obesity	BMI = 30.0 to 34.0
Major Obesity	BMI = 35.0 to 39.9
Morbid Obesity	BMI = 40.0 +

A BMI less than 18.5 is considered underweight and is associated with health risks

BMI = 18.5 to 24.5 is desirable and is associated with less health risks.

BMI = 25.0 to 27.0 is considered overweight; a caution zone; health risks for some people.

BMI = 27.1 to 29.9 is also considered overweight and is associated with health risks.

BMI greater or = 30.0 is defined as obesity; associated with increased health risks.

For those wishing to do without a lot of unnecessary mathematics, skip to the first text paragraph on page 61.

For those wishing to know more details, you may calculate your BMI as follows. Convert your weight in pounds to kilograms (kg) by dividing by 2.2. Convert your height in inches into centimeters (cm) by multiplying by 2.54 then, divide by 100 to convert to meters (m); or you may simply multiply inches by 0.0254 to convert directly to meters. Once you have calculated your height in meters for example 1.65, multiply it by the same number (1.65) to get the result in meters squared (m2), 2.72. Then, divide your weight in kg by this result.

Example: For a person (male or female) weighing 170 pounds and measuring 5 feet 5 inches tall.

Weight: 170 pounds divided by 2.2 = 77.3 kg

Height: 5'5" = 5 feet X 12 inches per foot + 5
inches = 65 inches

65 inches X 2.54 = 165 cm

165 cm divided by 100 = 1.65 meters

OR

65 inches X 0.0254 = 1.65 meters

Height in meters squared = 1.65 X 1.65 = 2.72 m2

BMI = weight in kg / height in m2

= 77.3 / 2.72 = **28**

The desirable body weight in this example is 111 to 147 pounds (BMI = 18.5 to 24.9). If using the table, simply look up columns 19 to 25 and the 5'5" row, which correspond to 114 to 150 pounds.

Adjusted Body Weight

Although muscle is metabolically active (burns calories), fat is not. Calculating estimated calorie needs using the entire weight of an obese person would over estimate these needs.

If you are overweight (have a BMI over 25) you can calculate you **adjusted weight** with the following equation. (You may choose to use your actual weight (in kg) for a BMI of less than 30).

(Current weight – desirable weight) X 0.25 + desirable weight

Subtract your desirable weight from your current weight. Desirable weight corresponds to the weight that would yield a BMI of 25 (or 24.9) based on your height.
Example: 170 – 147 pounds (using the upper end of the desirable range) = 23 pounds

Multiply this result by 0.25

Example: 23 pounds X 0.25 = 5.75 pounds

Add this result to your desirable weight (upper end of range)

Example: 5.75 + 147 pounds = **153 pounds** = **adjusted weight**

This adjusted weight should be used to estimate caloric needs in the calorie/kg and Harris Benedict equations. Your actual weight should be entered when entering data in the equations "for women and men of normal or excessive weight aged 19 and over." Consider consulting a Registered Dietitian if you find the mathematics to estimate caloric needs and to develop your meal plan too complicated.

Equations

There are different equations and methods to estimate daily caloric needs. One of the simplest methods is to use the **calories (kilocalories or kcal) per kg** method.

Sedentary   25 to 30 kcal/kg
Moderately active 35 kcal/kg
Very Active   40 kcal/kg

Example: with an adjusted weight of 153 pounds 69.5 kg (pounds are divided by 2.2)

Sedentary   25 to 30 kcal/kg
                      X   69.5 kg adjusted weight
                             1 739 to 2 086 calories

Moderately active   35 kcal/kg
                      X   69.5 kg adjusted weight
                             2 434 calories

Very Active   40 kcal/kg
                      X   69.5 kg adjusted weight
                             2 782 calories

This is the number of calories the individual in this example is estimated to burn per day. To lose weight, 300 to 500 calories per day should be subtracted.

Example: A moderately active person with an adjusted weight of 69.5 kg, hence estimated to burn 2434 calories per day, could start off with a diet providing approximately **1900 to 2100 calories**
2434 calories – **(300 to 500 calories)** = **1934 to 2134 calories**

Other Ways to Estimate Caloric Needs

For those wanting to be more precise by taking gender, height and age into account while estimating caloric needs, one of the following equations may be used:

For women aged 19 and over:
354 - (6.91 X age in years) + AF X (9.36 X weight in kg + 726 X height in meters)

AF = Activity factor: 1 if sedentary
1.12 if lightly active
1.27 if active
1.45 if very active

For men aged 19 and over:
662 - (9.53 X age in years) + AF X (15.91 X weight in kg + 539.6 X height in meters)

AF = Activity factor: 1 if sedentary
1.11 if lightly active
1.25 if active
1.48 if very active

For women of normal or excessive weight aged 19 and over:
387 - (7.31 X age in years) + AF X (10.9 X weight in kg + 660.7 X height in meters)

AF = Activity factor: 1 if sedentary
1.14 if lightly active
1.27 if active
1.45 if very active

For men of normal or excessive weight aged 19 and over:
864 - (9.72X age in years) + AF X (14.2 X weight in kg + 503 X height in meters)

AF = Activity factor: 1 if sedentary
                                   1.12 if lightly active
                                   1.27 if active
                                   1.45 if very active

Harris Benedict Equation:
Females: 665 + (9.6 X wt) + (1.8 X ht) – (4.7 X age)

Males: 66 + (13.7 X wt) + (5 X ht) – (6.8 X age)

wt: weight in kg, use adjusted weight if overweight
ht: height in cm
age: age in years

Example: A 35-year-old woman weighing 170 pounds, 5'5" tall
        Adjusted weight = 69.5 kg
        Height = 165 cm

Basal energy expenditure
~ 665 + (9.6 X 69.5 kg) + (1.8 X 165 cm) – (4.7 X 35 yrs.) = **1416 calories**

Now we have to multiply by an activity factor:
        Bed-bound: 1.2
        Sedentary (in a chair or able to walk): 1.3
        Activities of daily living: 1.5

Suppose this lady is sedentary. Use a factor of 1.3
        1416 X 1.3 = **1840 calories**

If she is quite active with household chores and does

many errands use a factor of 1.5

1416 X 1.5 = **2123 calories**

Subtract 300 to 500 calories form this result to determine the calorie level to promote **weight loss.**

1840 **– 300** = 1540 calories = **1500 calorie diet**

OR

2123 **– 500** = 1623 calories = **1600 calorie diet**

Now that you have estimated the number of calories you burn each day, **subtract 300 to 500 calories** from this amount to determine the appropriate calorie level **to promote weight loss**. Then, you will build a meal plan based on this calorie level. For instance, if you are a moderately active 36-year-old female and use the table on page 49 to estimate your calorie level, you are estimated to burn 2000 calories per day. In order to lose weight, your diet plan should be one of 1500 to 1700 calories (2000 minus 300 to 500 calories).

The lists of food exchanges (or portions) on the next page indicate the amount of calories per food group. By dividing your diet plan calorie allowance (for example 1700 calories) into sufficient portions of each food group to meet national food guide recommendations (see Appendices), you can calculate how many portions (exchanges) of each food group to eat each day to meet that calorie level. Next, divide the total food group portions into meals and snacks. Different combinations of portions per food group are possible to meet one given calorie level. See the **standard diet patterns** section for suggestions (pages 76 to 94). Depending on your needs (when you experience hypoglycemic symptoms or hunger), you could have one to three snacks per day (theoretically even more if you wished).

STARCHES: 80 calories per portion (exchange)

DAIRY PRODUCTS: 90 calories per portion of skim (fat-free); **100 calories** per portion of 1%; and **120 calories** per serving of 2% milk product. Avoid whole milk (150 calories per cup) and read labels on yogurt limiting to 120 calories per serving

VEGETABLES: 25 calories per portion

FRUIT: 60 calories per portion

MEAT AND SUBSTITUTES: Choose meats and substitutes with **35 to 75 calories** per ounce or 30 g (an exchange). Avoid those with 100 calories or more per ounce (30 g).

ADDED FATS: 45 calories per portion (exchange)

6- BUILDING YOUR PERSONALIZED MEAL PLAN

This chapter provides the necessary information to enable you to stay within your estimated caloric needs for weight loss, maintenance or weight gain, without actually counting the number of calories of every item you eat.

We will refer to **exchanges.** Exchanges are portion sizes of food items listed by category (starches, fruits, vegetables, milk products, meats or alternatives and fats). Each portion size listed within a category is approximately equal in calories.

Once you become familiar with exchange portions it will be easy to know how much food from each category meets the number of portions (exchanges) on your meal plan. Consider highlighting the items you want to choose most often. All portions of rice, pasta, cooked cereals (ex: oatmeal), meats and legumes (ex: chickpeas) should be measured after being cooked.

The most common portion is ½ cup (120 mL). Milk products are the exception however; a portion is equal to **1 cup (240 mL) of milk** (choose skim, 1% or 2%) or **¾ cup or 180 mL yogurt** (no more than 2% **M.F.**).
A **starch** portion is equal to **1 slice of bread (30 g or 1 oz)** for example; think one-half when choosing larger items: ½ English muffin, hamburger bun, hot dog bun, pita bread or small bagel. A portion of **cooked**

pasta, potato or corn is ½ **cup (120 ml)**. Don't worry, most plans allow for more than one starch per meal. If your plan allows for 2 starches at dinner and you feel like eating pasta, your portion should be 2 times (exchanges of) ½ cup totaling 1 cup (240 ml). If it allowed for 3 starches and you wanted **rice (⅓ cup or 80 mL per portion**), your portion should be 1 cup or 240 mL (3 X ⅓ cup or 3 X 80 mL)).

If you do not find a particular starch item (made from flour, rice, corn or potato) on the list provided, simply refer to the food label on the packaging to determine the portion that would provide approximately 80 calories. For instance, if a particular cereal lists one portion as 1 cup on the food label and that contains 200 calories, having half of the indicated amount on the label, ½ cup would yield 100 calories (approximately the equivalent of one starch exchange).

A **small- to medium-sized whole fruit** is generally considered a portion, or ½ **cup** unsweetened canned **fruit or juice**. If the item is large, once again think half: ½ a banana, grapefruit or mango. Small fruit such as plums can be doubled to 2 per portion. Examples of a portion or exchange are 1¼ cup (300 mL) strawberries or 15 grapes.

A simple way to estimate **vegetable** portions is **1 cup (240 mL) raw** or ½ **cup (120 mL) cooked vegetable**, **tomato sauce** or **vegetable juice**.

Meats and substitutes are generally counted by the **ounce (1 oz = 30 g)**. A pre-sliced slice of turkey luncheon meat is about 1 ounce (check label). One ounce of cheese (choose with no more than 15% M.F.) is about the size of a large dice or one-inch cube. A **3-ounce (90 g) portion of meat** is about the **size of a deck of cards**, whereas 3 ounces of **fish** fillet is the size of a **checkbook**. Other portions (exchanges) include **½ cup (120 mL) cooked dried bean, lentils or other legumes, 1 Tbsp (15 mL) nuts or seeds** or **1 egg**.

A **fat portion** is generally **1 tsp (5 mL)** of items such as **oil, margarine (choose non-hydrogenated), butter** (avoid) and **mayonnaise**. A portion of added fat is equal to **2 tsp (10 mL) of peanut butter** (try to buy non-hydrogenated), **⅛ avocado, 1 Tbsp (15 mL) salad dressing**, or **8 large olives**.

Your meal plan will indicate how many **exchanges** to have at each meal and snack. Refer to the lists below to learn the exchange measurements. Multiply this portion by the number of exchanges (or portions) you are to have at a given meal. The result is the amount of food you should put on your plate. Remember, all portions of grains, meats and alternatives should be measured after being cooked.

Metric Conversion

1 teaspoon (tsp) = 5 mL   1 ounce (oz) = 30 grams (g)
2 teaspoon (tsp) = 10 mL
1 tablespoon (Tbsp) = 15 mL

¼ cup = 60 mL   ½ cup = 120 mL   ⅔ cup = 160 mL
¾ cup = 180 mL   ⅓ cup = 80 mL   1 cup = 240 mL

Food Group Exchanges (Portions):

STARCHES (80 calories, 15 g of carbohydrates, 3 g of protein and a trace of fat per portion)

BREADS (30 g or 1 oz)

Bread	1 slice
Dinner roll (2")	1
Light or diet bread	2 slices
Bagel	½
English muffin	½
Hamburger bun	½
Hot dog bun	½
Pita bread (6"; 15 cm)	½
Tortilla	½

CRACKERS

Graham (2.5" square)	3
Melba Toast, oblong	4
Popcorn (non-fat)	3 cups
Pretzels	¾ oz (20 g)
Rice cakes	2
Wheat crackers	4
Soda crackers	6

CEREALS

Cooked (oatmeal, bulgur, cream of wheat)	½ cup
Dry, unsweetened cereals	¾ cup
Puffed wheat	1½ cups
Wheat germ, Grape Nuts	3 tsp
Corn meal, dry	2½ Tbsp
Pasta	½ cup
Rice	⅓ cup

PREPARED FOODS (1 starch+1 fat)

Biscuit, 2" diameter	1
Cornbread 2"x2"x1"	1
Chow mein noodles	½ cup
Potato chips (2 fats)	1 oz (30 g)

French fries, thin_____10 to 15
Stuffing_____¼ cup
Pancakes, 4" diameter_____2
Waffle, 5" X ½"_____1

STARCHY VEGETABLES
Corn_____1 ear or ½ cup
Baked beans_____⅓ cup
Potato_____1 small or ½ cup
Yam or sweet potato_____½ cup
Plantain_____½ cup
Winter squash_____1 cup
Pumpkin_____¾ cup

DESSERTS (occasionally)
Arrowroot, social tea cookies_____4
Gingerbread cookies_____3
Goglu™, Village™ or digestive cookies_____2
Granola (1 fat)_____¼ cup
Pudding, sugar-free_____½ cup
Ice cream (2 fats)_____½ cup
Ice milk (1 fat)_____½ cup
Sherbet_____¼ cup

SOUPS
Cream soup_____½ cup
Vegetable or chicken noodle_____1 cup

DAIRY PRODUCTS (90 to 120 calories, 12 g
carbohydrate, 8 g of protein and a trace to 5 g fat per
portion)

Evaporated skim milk_____½ cup
Enriched soy milk_____1 cup
Low fat buttermilk_____1 cup
Milk, skim, 1%, 2%_____1 cup
Non-fat dry milk_____⅓ cup
Yogurt_____¾ cup

VEGETABLES (25 calories, 5 g carbohydrate, 2 g protein per portion)
½ cup cooked or 1 cup raw
Count avocado and olives as a fat instead of a vegetable.

An extra 3 cups of the following vegetables are allowed in addition to those on your plan. They contain less than 20 calories per serving.

Celery	Cucumber	Spinach
Mushrooms	Green onion	Parsley
Cabbage	Endive	Radish
Alfalfa sprouts	Zucchini	

FRUIT (60 calories, 15 g carbohydrate per portion)

<u>FRESH FRUIT</u>

Apple (raw 2" diameter)	1
Orange (2½" diameter)	1
Peach	1
Pear	1 small
Kiwi (large)	1
Banana (9")	½
Grapefruit	½
Mango	½
Plums	2
Clementines	2
Figs (fresh)	2
Apricots (raw)	4
Cherries	12
Grapes (small)	15
Fruit salad	½ cup
Applesauce, unsweetened	½ cup
Blueberries	¾ cup
Pineapple (raw)	¾ cup
(canned)	⅓ cup
Papaya	1 cup
Raspberries	1 cup
Cubed, or honeydew	1 cup
Watermelon	1¼ cup
Strawberries	1¼ cup
Cantaloupe (5" diameter)	⅓ melon

FRUIT JUICE

Apple juice/cider_____	½ cup
Cranberry juice_____	⅓ cup
Cranberry juice, low calorie_____	1 cup
Grape juice_____	⅓ cup
Grapefruit juice_____	½ cup
Orange juice_____	½ cup

DRIED FRUIT

Raisins _____	2 Tbsp
Prunes_____	2
Dates_____	2½
Figs_____	1½
Apricots_____	7 halves

MEATS AND SUBSTITUTES

VERY LEAN MEATS AND SUBSTITUTES
(35 calories, no carbohydrates, 7 g protein, 0 to 1 g fat)

Poultry: Chicken or turkey (white meat,
   no skin), _____1 oz
Fish: Cod, sole, tilapia, flounder, haddock, halibut,
   trout, tuna (fresh or canned in water)_1 oz
Shellfish: Shrimp, lobster, scallops,
   clams, crab, imitation shellfish_____1 oz
Game: Pheasant (no skin), buffalo,
   venison, ostrich_____1 oz
Cheese with 1 g fat or less per oz:
   Nonfat or low-fat cheese_____1 oz
   Cottage cheese_____¼ cup
Other: Processed sandwich meats with 1 g of fat or less
   per oz, deli meats, turkey ham,
   chipped beef,_____1 oz
   Egg substitute, plain_____¼ cup
   Egg whites_____2
   Kidney (high cholesterol)_____1 oz
   Sausage or veggie dog with
   less than 1 g fat per oz_____1 oz

Count as 1 lean meat + 1 starch:
Legumes (dried beans,
split peas, lentils, chickpeas)_____½ cup

LEAN MEATS AND SUBSTITUTES
(55 calories, no carbohydrates, 7 g protein, 3 g fat)

Poultry: Chicken, turkey (dark meat no skin),
   chicken white meat with skin,
   domestic goose or duck
   (drained of fat, no skin)_____1 oz
Fish: Tuna (canned in oil, drained)_____1 oz
   Salmon (fresh or canned), catfish___1 oz
   Sardines (canned)_____2 medium
   Herring (smoked or uncreamed)____1 oz
   Oysters_____6 medium
Pork: Lean pork, fresh, canned, cured or
   boiled ham, tenderloin, center loin
   chop, Canadian bacon_____1 oz
Beef: Lean beef trimmed of fat,
   such as round, sirloin,
   tenderloin, flank steak,
   roast (rib. Chuck, rump),
   steak (porterhouse, T-bone,)
   ground round_____1 oz
Lamb: Chop, roast, leg_____1 oz
Game: Goose (no skin), rabbit_____1 oz
Veal: Lean chop, roast_____1 oz
Cheese: Cheese with 3 g
   of fat or less per oz_____1 oz
   4½% fat cottage cheese_____¼ cup
   Grated parmesan_____2 Tbsp
Other: Processed sandwich meat with
   3 g fat or less per serving
   example: turkey pastrami _____1 oz
   Hot dog with 3 g fat
   or less per oz_____1½ oz
   Liver, heart (high cholesterol)_____1 oz

MEDIUM-FAT MEATS AND SUBSTITUTES
(75 calories, no carbohydrates, 7 g protein, 5 g fat)

Poultry: Dark chicken meat (with skin),
ground chicken or turkey,
fried chicken (with skin)_____1 oz
Fish: Any fried fish_____1 oz
Pork: chop, cutlet, top loin, _____1 oz
Beef: Most beef cuts (ground beef, prime rib,
meatloaf, short ribs, corned beef)____1 oz
Lamb: Rib roast, ground_____1 oz
Veal: Cutlet (un-breaded cubed
or ground)_____1 oz
Cheese: With 5 g of fat or less per oz
Mozzarella_____1 oz
Feta_____1 oz
Ricotta_____¼ cup
Other: Egg limit to 2 per week if on cardiac
diet, otherwise maximum 1/day____1
Tempeh_____¼ cup
Tofu_____4 oz or ½ cup
Sausage (5 g fat or less per oz)_____1 oz

HIGH-FAT MEATS AND SUBSTITUTES
(100 calories, no carbohydrates, 7 g protein, 8 g fat)
Choose from this list occasionally if at all.

Pork: Ground pork, pork sausage,
Spareribs_____1 oz
Cheese: All regular cheeses, cheddar, Swiss,
American, Monterey Jack_____1 oz
Other: Processed sandwich meats with 8 g of
fat per oz or less, bologna, salami___1 oz
Bacon (20 slices/lb) _____3 slices
Hot dog (chicken or turkey)_____1 (10/lb)
Sausage, Italian, Polish, smoked____1 oz
*Counts as one high-fat meat + one fat
exchange (**try to avoid**):*
Hot dog (beef or pork)_____1 (10/lb)

ADDED FATS (45 calories, 5 g fat)

MONOUNSATURATED FATS *Choose often*

Oil (olive, canola, peanut)	1 tsp (5 mL)
Tahini paste	1 tsp (5 mL)
Peanut butter	2 tsp (10 mL)
Sesame seeds	1 Tbsp (15 mL)
Nuts: Pecans	4 halves
Cashews, almonds	6 nuts
Mixed	6 nuts
Peanuts	10 nuts
Avocado	⅛ (1 oz)
Olives: Black	8 large
Stuffed green	10 large

POLYUNSATURATED FATS

Margarine (choose non-hydrogenated)	1 tsp (5 mL)
Light margarine	1 Tbsp (15 mL)
Mayonnaise: regular	1 tsp (5 mL)
low-fat	1 Tbsp (15 mL)
Miracle Whip Salad Dressing™:	
regular	2 tsp (10 mL)
Reduced-fat	1 Tbsp (15 mL)
Oil (safflower, corn, soybean)	1 tsp (5 mL)
Salad dressing: regular	1 Tbsp (15 mL)
low-fat	2 Tbsp (30 mL)
Nuts, walnuts	4 halves
Seeds: sunflower, pumpkin	1 Tbsp (15 mL)

SATURATED FATS *Avoid except for reduced-fat cream cheese and sour cream*

Butter:	1 tsp (5 mL)
whipped	2 tsp (10 mL)
Cream cheese: regular	1 Tbsp (15 mL), ½ oz
reduced-fat	2 Tbsp (60 mL), 1 oz
Coconut	2 Tbsp (30 mL)
Cream (half and half)	2 Tbsp (30 mL)
Sour cream: regular	2 Tbsp (30 mL)
low-fat	3 Tbsp (45 mL)

Bacon_____	1 slice
	(20 slices/lb)
Chitterlings, boiled_____	2 Tbsp (30 mL),
	½ oz
Salt pork, fatback or_____	¼ oz
Lard or shortening_____	1 tsp (5 mL)

It's a little tricky at first to "guesstimate" portions of combined food items, such as a casserole, pizza or lasagna. It will get easier to eyeball a serving and have in mind how many portions it contains. For example, a piece of lasagna made of pasta, meat sauce and cheese. Does it have less meat than the size of a deck of cards, and 1 or 2 oz of cheese? How many half-cups of pasta are in the portion?

One-half of a 10" thin pizza (three slices) with cold cuts and cheese is approximately the equivalent of 3 starches, 3 meats and 1 fat; the same portion of a thick crust pizza would correspond to 5 starches and 4 meats.

Any diabetic exchange list can assist you in learning portion sizes. They can be found in some diabetic cookbooks, medical clinics and can be purchased on the website of the American Diabetic Association at *http://store.diabetes.org/*. Simply enter the word exchanges in the search box and select *Exchange List for Weight Management (single)*.

Now that you have information on the calorie levels of the different food groups, practice reading labels. A PRIA™ bar for example, containing 170 calories, 10 grams of protein and 6 grams of fat per serving. This would correspond closely to a starch plus a meat exchange (starch with 80 calories, 3 g of protein, meat with 75 calories, 7 g of protein and 5 g of fat) and would provide a total of 155 calories, 7 g of protein and 5 g of fat. Don't fret over the 15-calorie difference. The plan is based on averages and approximations.

Be aware that the nutritional information on a food label ("Nutrition Facts") reflects the amount of nutrients in one serving — that is the portion determined by the manufacturer which may differ from the portions in your meal plan. Try to respect the portions in your meal plan.

Now you are ready to build your meal plan. Divide your calorie allowance (see Chapter 5 – *Estimating Caloric Needs*), the result of your estimated calorie needs minus 300 to 500 calories to lose weight, into portions (exchanges) of the various food groups among your preferred daily meals and snacks pattern (example: 3 meals and 3 snacks/day). If you don't want to figure out your own meal pattern, select a standard diet pattern from the following examples corresponding to your estimated caloric needs for weight loss (or for weight maintenance if your goal is to maintain your current weight).

If you choose to design you own meal plan, refer to the appendices (Appendix 1- *Canada's Food Guide* or Appendix 2- *U.S. 2005 Revised Dietary Guidelines*). Another option is to log-on to *www.mypyramid.gov* to obtain a customized calorie-level meal plan based on your age, gender and activity level. Remember to subtract 300 to 500 calories for weight loss.

I have only included two servings of dairy products in the standard meal patterns of less than 1400 calories. This meets Canada's Food Guide recommendations. If you want to include more dairy products, as suggested in the Revised U.S. Guidelines, either add another portion of dairy and subtract either a starch or meat exchange, or have 2 ounces of low-fat cheese as a meat substitute.

The following pages include meal pattern examples corresponding to various calorie levels. You may design your own or chose from the standard diet patterns according to your estimated calorie level. Use it and then divide the indicated number of portions into your meal plan by filling out the blank form provided on page 97.

STANDARD DIET PATTERNS

1200 calories

	Number of Portions	Total Calories
STARCHES: **80 calories**/portion	5	400
DAIRY PRODUCTS: **90 calories**/portion (0%) **100 calories**/portion (1%) **120 calories/**portion (2%)	2	180
VEGETABLES: **25 calories**/portion	3	75
FRUIT: **60 calories**/portion	2	120
MEAT AND SUBST.: **75 calories**/portion (average)	5	375
ADDED FATS: **45 calories**/portion	2	<u>90</u>
TOTAL CALORIES		1240

1300 calories

	Number of Portions	Total Calories
STARCHES: **80 calories**/portion	5	400
DAIRY PRODUCTS: **90 calories**/portion (0%) **100 calories**/portion (1%) **120 calories/**portion (2%)	2	180
VEGETABLES: **25 calories**/portion	4	100
FRUIT: **60 calories**/portion	2	120
MEAT AND SUBST.: **75 calories**/portion (average)	5	375
ADDED FATS: **45 calories**/portion	3	<u>135</u>
TOTAL CALORIES		1310

1400 calories

	Number of Portions	Total Calories
STARCHES: **80 calories**/portion	6	480
DAIRY PRODUCTS: **90 calories**/portion (0%) **100 calories**/portion (1%) **120 calories/**portion (2%)	2	180
VEGETABLES: **25 calories**/portion	2	50
FRUIT: **60 calories**/portion	3	180
MEAT AND SUBST.: **75 calories**/portion (average)	5	375
ADDED FATS: **45 calories**/portion	3	<u>135</u>
TOTAL CALORIES		1400

1500 calories

	Number of Portions	Total Calories
STARCHES: **80 calories**/portion	6	480
DAIRY PRODUCTS: **90 calories**/portion (0%) **100 calories**/portion (1%) **120 calories/**portion (2%)	3	270
VEGETABLES: **25 calories**/portion	2	50
FRUIT: **60 calories**/portion	3	180
MEAT AND SUBST.: **75 calories**/portion (average)	5	375
ADDED FATS: **45 calories**/portion	3	<u>135</u>
TOTAL CALORIES		1490

1600 calories

	Number of Portions	Total Calories
STARCHES: 80 **calories**/portion	7	560
DAIRY PRODUCTS: 90 **calories**/portion (0%) 100 **calories**/portion (1%) 120 **calories/**portion (2%)	3	270
VEGETABLES: 25 **calories**/portion	2	50
FRUIT: 60 **calories**/portion	3	180
MEAT AND SUBST.: 75 **calories**/portion (average)	6	450
ADDED FATS: 45 **calories**/portion	3	<u>135</u>
TOTAL CALORIES		1645 calories

1700 calories

	Number of Portions	Total Calories
STARCHES: 80 calories/portion	7	560
DAIRY PRODUCTS: 90 calories/portion (0%) 100 calories/portion (1%) 120 calories/portion (2%)	3	270
VEGETABLES: 25 calories/portion	3	75
FRUIT: 60 calories/portion	4	240
MEAT AND SUBST.: 75 calories/portion (average)	6	450
ADDED FATS: 45 calories/portion	3	<u>135</u>
TOTAL CALORIES		1730

1800 calories

	Number of Portions	Total Calories
STARCHES: 80 **calories**/portion	8	640
DAIRY PRODUCTS: 90 **calories**/portion (0%) 100 **calories**/portion (1%) 120 **calories/**portion (2%)	3	270
VEGETABLES: 25 **calories**/portion	5	100
FRUIT: 60 **calories**/portion	3	180
MEAT AND SUBST.: 75 **calories**/portion (average)	6	450
ADDED FATS: 45 **calories**/portion	3	<u>135</u>
TOTAL CALORIES		1800

1900 calories

	Number of Portions	Total Calories
STARCHES: **80 calories**/portion	8	640
DAIRY PRODUCTS: **90 calories**/portion (0%) **100 calories**/portion (1%) **120 calories/**portion (2%)	3	270
VEGETABLES: **25 calories**/portion	5	125
FRUIT: **60 calories**/portion	4	240
MEAT AND SUBST.: **75 calories**/portion (average)	6	450
ADDED FATS: **45 calories**/portion	4	<u>180</u>
TOTAL CALORIES		1905

2000 calories

	Number of Portions	Total Calories
STARCHES: **80 calories**/portion	8	640
DAIRY PRODUCTS: **90 calories**/portion (0%) **100 calories**/portion (1%) **120 calories/**portion (2%)	3	270
VEGETABLES: **25 calories**/portion	5	125
FRUIT: **60 calories**/portion	4	240
MEAT AND SUBST.: **75 calories**/portion (average)	7	525
ADDED FATS: **45 calories**/portion	5	<u>225</u>
TOTAL CALORIES		2025

2100 calories

	Number of Portions	Total Calories
STARCHES: 80 **calories**/portion	9	720
DAIRY PRODUCTS: 90 **calories**/portion (0%) 100 **calories**/portion (1%) 120 **calories/**portion (2%)	3	270
VEGETABLES: 25 **calories**/portion	5	125
FRUIT: 60 **calories**/portion	4	240
MEAT AND SUBST.: 75 **calories**/portion (average)	7	525
ADDED FATS: 45 **calories**/portion	5	225
TOTAL CALORIES		2105

2200 calories

	Number of Portions	Total Calories
STARCHES: **80 calories**/portion	9	720
DAIRY PRODUCTS: **90 calories**/portion (0%) **100 calories**/portion (1%) **120 calories/**portion (2%)	3	270
VEGETABLES: **25 calories**/portion	5	125
FRUIT: **60 calories**/portion	4	240
MEAT AND SUBST.: **75 calories**/portion (average)	8	600
ADDED FATS: **45 calories**/portion	5	<u>225</u>
TOTAL CALORIES		2180

2300 calories

	Number of Portions	Total Calories
STARCHES: **80 calories**/portion	10	800
DAIRY PRODUCTS: **90 calories**/portion (0%) **100 calories**/portion (1%) **120 calories/**portion (2%)	3	270
VEGETABLES: **25 calories**/portion	5	125
FRUIT: **60 calories**/portion	4	240
MEAT AND SUBST.: **75 calories**/portion (average)	8	600
ADDED FATS: **45 calories**/portion	6	<u>270</u>
TOTAL CALORIES		2305

2400 calories

	Number of Portions	Total Calories
STARCHES: **80 calories**/portion	10	800
DAIRY PRODUCTS: **90 calories**/portion (0%) **100 calories**/portion (1%) **120 calories/**portion (2%)	4	400
VEGETABLES: **25 calories**/portion	5	125
FRUIT: **60 calories**/portion	4	240
MEAT AND SUBST.: **75 calories**/portion (average)	8	600
ADDED FATS: **45 calories**/portion	5	<u>225</u>
TOTAL CALORIES		2390

2500 calories

	Number of Portions	Total Calories
STARCHES: **80 calories**/portion	10	800
DAIRY PRODUCTS: **90 calories**/portion (0%) **100 calories**/portion (1%) **120 calories/**portion (2%)	4	400
VEGETABLES: **25 calories**/portion	5	125
FRUIT: **60 calories**/portion	5	300
MEAT AND SUBST.: **75 calories**/portion (average)	8	600
ADDED FATS: **45 calories**/portion	6	<u>270</u>
TOTAL CALORIES		2495

2600 calories

	Number of Portions	Total Calories
STARCHES: 80 **calories**/portion	11	880
DAIRY PRODUCTS: 90 **calories**/portion (0%) 100 **calories**/portion (1%) 120 **calories**/portion (2%)	4	400
VEGETABLES: 25 **calories**/portion	5	125
FRUIT: 60 **calories**/portion	4	240
MEAT AND SUBST.: 75 **calories**/portion (average)	9	675
ADDED FATS: 45 **calories**/portion	6	270
TOTAL CALORIES		2590

2700 calories

	Number of Portions	Total Calories
STARCHES: **80 calories**/portion	11	880
DAIRY PRODUCTS: **90 calories**/portion (0%) **100 calories**/portion (1%) **120 calories/**portion (2%)	4	480
VEGETABLES: **25 calories**/portion	5	125
FRUIT: **60 calories**/portion	4	240
MEAT AND SUBST.: **75 calories**/portion (average)	9	675
ADDED FATS: **45 calories**/portion	6	<u>270</u>
TOTAL CALORIES		2670

2800 calories

	Number of Portions	Total Calories
STARCHES: **80 calories**/portion	11	880
DAIRY PRODUCTS: **90 calories**/portion (0%) **100 calories**/portion (1%) **120 calories/**portion (2%)	4	480
VEGETABLES: **25 calories**/portion	5	125
FRUIT: **60 calories**/portion	5	300
MEAT AND SUBST.: **75 calories**/portion (average)	9	675
ADDED FATS: **45 calories**/portion	7	<u>315</u>
TOTAL CALORIES		2775

2900 calories

	Number of Portions	Total Calories
STARCHES: **80 calories**/portion	12	960
DAIRY PRODUCTS: **90 calories**/portion (0%) **100 calories**/portion (1%) **120 calories/**portion (2%)	4	480
VEGETABLES: **25 calories**/portion	5	125
FRUIT: **60 calories**/portion	6	300
MEAT AND SUBST.: **75 calories**/portion (average)	9	675
ADDED FATS: **45 calories**/portion	8	<u>360</u>
TOTAL CALORIES		2900

3000 calories

	Number of Portions	Total Calories
STARCHES: **80 calories**/portion	12	960
DAIRY PRODUCTS: **90 calories**/portion (0%) **100 calories**/portion (1%) **120 calories/**portion (2%)	4	480
VEGETABLES: **25 calories**/portion	5	125
FRUIT: **60 calories**/portion	6	360
MEAT AND SUBST.: **75 calories**/portion (average)	10	750
ADDED FATS: **45 calories**/portion	8	<u>360</u>
TOTAL CALORIES		3035

Now that you have determined the number of portions of each food group to eat, divide them among your meals and snacks on *YOUR MEAL PLAN* on page 97. Try to choose most of the food groups at each meal and try to include a carbohydrate choice (either a starch, fruit or dairy product) with protein (meat or substitutes, or dairy product) and/or added fat with snacks to slow digestion and keep you from feeling hungry sooner than necessary.

Fill in the blank meal plan page with your calorie level and the number of portions per meal and snacks. Use a pencil to allow for corrections. Build your own plan, choose from the preceding "standard diet patterns" or use one that has been calculated for you on-line at www.mypyramid.gov. Keep it within reach. Write down food portion examples for one typical day. Refer to examples on pages 98 to 102 for ideas. You are not restricted to the particular foods in the examples. Choose any foods in the appropriate amounts per category (group) according to your calorie level meal plan. Make a few days of menu examples with foods you enjoy on loose sheets of paper. This is an important learning exercise to help you put the information into practice. You can then keep your examples for quick reference when you don't have time to look up exchange portions on the lists before mealtime. You may interchange any lunch example you made up using your meal plan, because they contain the same number of exchanges each day, therefore are equal in calories. You may also interchange any breakfast or dinner examples. You get to choose the foods you would like to eat from the lists provided to make up your own meal plan. Measure each item accurately (with measuring cup and measuring spoons) the first two times you choose a new item. With repetition, you should have a good enough idea of portion sizes of the different food groups to "guesstimate", and be able to eventually set the meal plan aside, only referring to it to refresh your memory. Don't be too hard on yourself if you "indulge" a little. After all, we are not computers that can be programmed to eat in a constant manner. Enjoy, and then try to get back on track.

You may consult a cookbook with the "diabetic exchanges" (the same ones used here) for convenient ideas of recipes to coincide with your meal plan portions. Some specialize in meals that can be prepared in less than 30 minutes. Such cookbooks are available on the website of the American Diabetic Association at http://store.diabetes.org/. Click on *Cookbooks*, then on *Quick and Easy Cooking*. The website of the Canadian Diabetic Association at www.diabetes.ca/literature/ offers a selection of cookbooks; click *on Literature Order Form*. For French recipes, try www.diabete.qc.ca/, click *on livres de recettes. La nouvelle cuisine santé* by Poissant-Laurin, Raymond and Rouette, Edition Stanké, uses the exchanges.

If you still feel hungry after eating the portions the meal plan provides without skipping meals or snacks containing **carbohydrates**, **protein** and **fat**, by all means, EAT! You should not let yourself get too hungry, otherwise you are not likely to stick to the plan. Choose extra items that score high on the **satiety index** (pages 43 to 44). If you eat more in one day, you are likely to feel less hungry the next, and better able to stick to the plan. The first week is the most difficult. No one wants to be restricted to a pattern. Tell yourself this is temporary until you learn the average portions to eat in a day and are able to gage your intake from then on. Think of it as a learning tool to practice portioning meals and snacks, and to remind you to get all the necessary food groups in, instead of a rigid diet.

YOUR MEAL PLAN: _____ calories

 # Exchanges/
Food Group   **Serving Size**   **Food**

BREAKFAST__AM/PM

_____Starches   _____   _____
_____Fruit   _____   _____
_____Milk product   _____   _____
_____Meat or subst.   _____   _____
_____Added Fat   _____   _____

AM SNACK___AM/PM

_____   _____   _____
_____   _____   _____
_____   _____   _____

LUNCH_____AM/PM

_____Starches   _____   _____
_____Fruit   _____   _____
_____Vegetables   _____   _____
_____Milk product   _____   _____
_____Meat or subst.   _____   _____
_____Added Fat   _____   _____

PM SNACK___AM/PM

_____   _____   _____
_____   _____   _____
_____   _____   _____

DINNER:_____AM/PM

_____Starches   _____   _____
_____Fruit   _____   _____
_____Vegetables   _____   _____
_____Milk product   _____   _____
_____Meat or subst.   _____   _____
_____Added Fat   _____   _____

EVENING SNACK____AM/PM

_____   _____   _____
_____   _____   _____

Example of 1700-calorie meal plan using a standard pattern from pages 76 to 94.

YOUR MEAL PLAN: _1700_ calories

 # Exchanges/
Food Group   **Serving Size**   **Food**

BREAKFAST__7 AM

2____Starches   _____   _____
1____Fruit   _____   _____
1____Milk product   _____   _____
____Meat or subst._____   _____
1____Added Fat   _____   _____

AM SNACK____10 AM

1____fruit__   _____   _____
1____milk__   _____   _____

LUNCH_noon_PM

2____Starches   _____   _____
1____Fruit   _____   _____
1____Vegetables   _____   _____
____Milk product   _____   _____
2____Meat or subst._____   _____
1____Added Fat   _____   _____

PM SNACK____3 PM

1____starch__   _____   _____
1____meat__   _____   _____

DINNER:____6 PM

1____Starches   _____   _____
1____Fruit   _____   _____
2____Vegetables   _____   _____
½____Milk product   _____   _____
3____Meat or subst._____   _____
1____Added Fat   _____   _____

EVENING SNACK____8 PM

1____starch__   _____   _____
½____milk__   _____   _____

Example of 1700 calorie meal plan using a standard pattern from pages 76 to 94.

YOUR MEAL PLAN: <u>1700</u> calories

# Exchanges/ Food Group	Serving Size	Food
BREAKFAST 7 AM		
2 Starches	1	English muffin
1 Fruit	1½	banana
1 Milk product	8 oz	skim milk
___ Meat or subst.		
1 Added Fat	2tsp	peanut-butter
AM SNACK 10 AM		
1 fruit	1	orange
1 milk	¾ cup	yogurt
LUNCH noon PM		
2 Starches	2	2 slices bread (whole grain)
1 Fruit	15	grapes
1 Vegetables	1 cup	raw veggies
___ Milk product		
2 Meat or subst.	2 oz	turkey
1 Added Fat	1 tsp	mayonnaise
PM SNACK 3 PM		
1 starch	4	Melba Toast
1 meat	1 oz	cheese
DINNER: 6 PM		
1 Starches	½ cup	mashed potato
1 Fruit	1¼ cup	strawberries
2 Vegetables	2 cups	salad
½ Milk product	4 oz	skim milk
3 Meat or subst.	3 oz	salmon
1 Added Fat	1 Tbs	salad dressing
EVENING SNACK 8 PM		
1 starch	¾ cup	dry cereal
½ milk	4 oz	skim milk

Example of 1400 calorie meal plan using a standard pattern from pages 76 to 94.

YOUR MEAL PLAN: <u>1400</u> calories

# Exchanges/ Food Group	Serving Size	Food
BREAKFAST__7 AM		
1____Starches	1	English muffin
1____Fruit	½	banana
½____Milk product	4 oz	skim milk
____Meat or subst.		
1____Added Fat	2tsp	peanut-butter
AM SNACK____10 AM		
1____fruit	1	orange
½____milk	½ cup	yogurt
LUNCH____noon PM		
2____Starches	2	2 slices bread (whole grain)
____Fruit		
1____Vegetables	1 cup	raw veggies
____Milk product		
2____Meat or subst.	2 oz	turkey
1____Added Fat	1 tsp	mayonnaise
PM SNACK____3 PM		
1____starch	4	Melba Toast
1____meat	1 oz	cheese
DINNER:____6 PM		
1____Starches	½ cup	mashed potato
1____Fruit	1¼ cup	strawberries
1____Vegetables	1 cups	salad
½____Milk product	4 oz	skim milk
2____Meat or subst.	2 oz	salmon
1____Added Fat	1 Tbs	salad dressing
EVENING SNACK____8 PM		
1____starch	¾ cup	dry cereal
½____milk	4 oz	skim milk

Building Your Personalized Meal Plan -- 101

YOUR MEAL PLAN: <u>2000</u> calories

# Exchanges/ Food Group	Serving Size	Food
BREAKFAST__7 AM		
2____Starches	1	English muffin
1____Fruit	1/2	banana
1____Milk product	8 oz	skim milk
1____Meat or subst.	1	egg
1____Added Fat	2 tsp.	peanut-butter
AM SNACK____10 AM		
1____fruit	1	orange
1____milk	¾ cup	yogurt
LUNCH_noon_PM		
2____Starches	2	2 slices bread (whole grain)
1____Fruit	15	grapes
2____Vegetables	2 cups	raw veggies
____Milk product		
2____Meat or subst.	2 oz	turkey
1____Added Fat	1 tsp	mayonnaise
PM SNACK____3 PM		
1____starch	4	Melba Toast
1____meat	1 oz	cheese
1____Added Fat	6	almonds
DINNER:____6 PM		
2____Starches	1 cup	mashed potato
1____Fruit	1¼ cup	strawberries
3____Vegetables	1½ cups	cooked veggies
½____Milk product	4 oz	skim milk
3____Meat or subst.	3 oz	salmon
2____Added Fat	2 Tbs	salad dressing
EVENING SNACK____8 PM		
1____starch	¾ cup	dry cereal
½____milk	4 oz	skim milk

YOUR MEAL PLAN: <u>2300</u> calories

 # Exchanges/
Food Group	Serving Size	Food
BREAKFAST__7 AM		
2____Starches	1	English muffin
1____Fruit	½	banana
1____Milk product	8 oz	skim milk
1____Meat or subst.	1	egg
1____Added Fat	2tsp	peanut-butter
AM SNACK____10 AM		
1____fruit	1	orange
1____milk	¾ cup	yogurt
LUNCH_noon_PM		
2____Starches	2	2 slices bread (whole grain)
1____Fruit	15	grapes
2____Vegetables	2 cups	raw veggies
____Milk product		
3____Meat or subst.	3 oz	turkey
2____Added Fat	2 tsp	mayonnaise
PM SNACK____3 PM		
1____starch	1	Melba Toast
1____meat	1 oz	cheese
1____Added Fat	6	almonds
DINNER:____6 PM		
3____Starches	½ cup	mashed potato
1____Fruit	1¼ cup	strawberries
3____Vegetables	1½ cup	cooked veggies
½____Milk product	4 oz	skim milk
3____Meat or subst.	3 oz	salmon
2____Added Fat	1 Tbs	salad dressing
EVENING SNACK____8 PM		
2____starch	1½ cup	dry cereal
½____milk	4 oz	skim milk

7- FOOD JOURNAL

You may consider writing down what and when you eat, as well as how you feel. Even if you do this for only for 3 consecutive days (including one weekend day), it can be a useful tool to indicate when/if meals or snacks have been missed, or if meals were more than five hours apart, and whether this resulted or not in any of the hypoglycemic symptoms mentioned (see Chapter 1 - *What is Hypoglycemia?*). Try writing down what and when you eat on the following three pages, as well as how you feel after starting this proposed eating plan. See if you feel better and more in control of your appetite.

Make it a rule to only eat at the kitchen, dining room or patio table. If you are really hungry for another snack, you may have one, but must feel hungry enough to be willing to interrupt your television viewing to sit in the kitchen. Turn off the television and do not read while eating. Like Pavlov's dog, we may begin to associate watching television with eating, and develop the urge to eat every time we are watching television. Watching television or reading while eating distracts us from the pleasure of eating. We may not feel as satisfied, not have had the "conscious" pleasure of eating and therefore be more prone to want to eat again.

FOOD JOURNAL (choose three consecutive days)

	Day #1 date:	Foods eaten and quantities	Symptoms
Breakfast	time:		
AM Snack	time:		
Lunch	time:		
PM Snack	time:		
Dinner	time:		
Evening Snack	time:		

FOOD JOURNAL (choose three consecutive days)

	Day #2 date:	Foods eaten and quantities	symptoms
Breakfast	time:		
AM Snack	time:		
Lunch	time:		
PM Snack	time:		
Dinner	time:		
Evening Snack	time:		

FOOD JOURNAL (choose three consecutive days)

	Day #3 date:	Foods eaten and quantities	symptoms
Breakfast	time:		
AM Snack	time:		
Lunch	time:		
PM Snack	time:		
Dinner	time:		
Evening Snack	time:		

You may consider completing the 3-day food journal only after you have reviewed the food portions in each group, made up 3 menu examples and measured new food items the first 2 times eaten. Does doing all the above at the same time feel overwhelming? If that is the case, only start the food journal 2 or 3 weeks into the program. This will make it easier to record your intake once you are more familiar with the portions. Take your time; there is no need to rush your learning. Some people chose to make changes gradually, 1 or 2 at a time. That is ok as well.

Don't quit now! You have just learned the most complicated sections of the program.

8- HOW EXERCISE AFFECTS BLOOD SUGAR

The revised *2005 Dietary Guidelines* for Americans include recommendations of a minimum of 30 minutes a day of moderate-to-vigorous activity, 60 minutes a day for most adults to avoid weight gain, 60 to 90 minutes a day to lose weight. Moderate-to-vigorous activities can include activities that increase respiration and heart rate during which you are still able to talk without feeling overly winded. Moderate-type exercises include walking (15 to 20 minute/mile; if your respiration is increased at a slower pace than this, it may be considered moderate or vigorous to you), cycling for pleasure and golfing without a cart. Sports play such as aerobics, running, basketball or soccer is considered vigorous. Light housework, light gardening or walking for pleasure are considered low intensity activities.

As mentioned in Chapter 5- *Estimating Caloric Needs*, be sure to include a resistance-type exercise a few times per week. Doing so can limit lean tissue loss. If you only do aerobic-type exercise such as walking or running, you are likely to breakdown muscle at some point to convert it to carbohydrate while you are dieting. This would lead to a lower **metabolic rate**. This in turn could lead to a "plateau", stagnant weight loss or even gaining weight on the same number of calories that once allowed you to maintain your weight. Your metabolic rate would be increased during the aerobic activity and for a short time afterwards, but be reduced the rest of the day. However, doing weight-bearing exercises increases metabolic rate 24 hours per day and burns more calories all day long, even while you sleep. Consider weight-training, floor exercises using your own body weight such as push-ups and lunges, Pilates, rubber band exercises, etc. Include exercises that target your large muscle groups such as thighs, back and chest. Be sure to get the approval of your doctor before starting an exercise program. To learn how to exercise safely or if you are limited by a physical condition, seek the assistance of a certified fitness trainer or physical therapist.

Whether you are an athlete or a casual exerciser 3 to 6 days per week, putting in 1 or more hours per workout, you may find the following information helpful.

The body primarily relies on fuel from carbohydrate and fat during exercise. The ratio of calories provided by carbohydrates and fat depends on the intensity of the exercise and how trained the athlete is. Even if an activity burns a greater percentage of calories from carbohydrates, a deficit in calories will cause fat stores to be tapped into post-workout to balance demand.

Carbohydrate is stored in the form of glycogen in the liver and muscles. When we fast, such as overnight, much of our glycogen stores in our liver are depleted. When we exercise, especially intensely and over long periods, stored muscle glycogen can run out. Because there may no longer be a steady supply of carbohydrate fuel led into the bloodstream (low blood sugar) and feeding the brain, fatigue, trouble concentrating or exhaustion could set in (see hypoglycemic symptoms in Chapter 1- *What is hypoglycemia?*).

This is why it is important to eat breakfast before a morning workout. Even if your muscles still hold glycogen, your liver could be depleted. This could sabotage your workout plans. The same rule applies when exercising more than 3 to 4 hours after eating; you may need a snack before your workout.

It is also important to eat carbohydrate soon after a workout. Waiting more than two hours post-workout to refuel glycogen stores can limit their repletion.

Carbohydrate: To Fuel Exercise

- Carbohydrate is the main source of fuel during exercise (from blood glucose and muscle glycogen). Sources from blood glucose can originate from food being absorbed, glycogen stores in the liver, or the body converting protein to carbohydrate.
- Carbohydrate enables one to workout longer and prevent hypoglycemia.
- Athletes will experience reduced endurance, fatigue and exhaustion once glycogen stores are depleted.
- Muscle glycogen depletion occurs during marathon-type events. Depletion can also occur during tournaments, or repeated training sessions over several days without adequate replacement with dietary carbohydrates or rest.
- Carbohydrate-rich foods are needed to replenish glycogen stores.
- Carbohydrates have a protein sparing effect; if insufficient sources of carbohydrate are available, protein, including muscle, is converted to carbohydrates to provide fuel during exercise.
- A high-carbohydrate meal eaten within two hours of exercising can increase glycogen storage by 300% (ex: orange juice and crackers)

- Carbohydrates are less "fattening'. Converting dietary fat to body fat requires only 3% of eaten calories, but converting dietary carbohydrates to body fat requires 23% of eaten calories.
- Eating mainly fat and protein decreases performance and leads to breakdown of tissue protein, hence muscle loss. Lean tissue loss decreases **metabolic rate**.

How Much Carbohydrate?

Most athletes need at least 8 servings of grain products, fruit and vegetables each day in order to maintain an adequate energy level. Endurance athletes (marathon runners, cyclists, tri-athletes) can eat 15 or more servings from these groups. When calorie intake is monitored, such as in gymnastics or diving, a minimum of 5 servings should be eaten. Refer to your personalized meal plan, based on your caloric needs to determine the number of portions you need.

The Best Carbohydrate Choices

"Complex" carbohydrates (bread, pasta, rice, cereal, legumes, starchy vegetables and fruit) are preferred over "simple" carbohydrates (sugar, candy, soda, except during or immediately after an event). They are richer in nutrients. If you can't resist concentrated sweets such as fat-free candy (jelly beans, jujubes, etc.), have a small portion soon after working out. Rapidly absorbed sugar can be beneficial in replenishing glycogen quickly. Beware of the calories you are adding to your meal plan by doing so.

To Maximize Muscle Glycogen Stores

- Muscle glycogen stores take **24 to 48 hours to replete** after intense exercise. Include rest days after hard training or prior to competitions and eat adequate amounts of carbohydrates to ensure maximum repletion of glycogen stores.

- Eat or drink high carbohydrate foods within the first 15 minutes after a competition or an intense workout. Eat frequent high-carbohydrate snacks during the 2 to 4 hours following exercise (fruit, yogurt, crackers, bagels, etc.)
- A carbohydrate-protein combination consumed immediately after intense exercise may be more effective in replenishing glycogen stores than carbohydrates alone. Try chocolate milk, tuna sandwich or fruit with yogurt.

What about "Sport Drinks"?

Plain cool water is sufficient for events lasting no more than **1 hour**.

Drinks made of 2½ to 10% carbohydrate are beneficial for activities lasting **more than 1 hour**. Look for drinks with 6 g of carbohydrates (glucose, glucose polymer or sucrose) per 100 mL of beverage. The addition of a small amount of **sodium** enhances carbohydrate absorption. You can make your own beverage by mixing unsweetened orange juice and water 50:50. **Try it first in training!**

Pre-Event Meals

Eat a high-carbohydrate, low fat and protein meal 2 to 3 hours before a competition. Protein and fat take longer to digest. Fluid should be consumed with the meal. Avoid gas-forming or unfamiliar foods and alcohol.

Examples:
Cereal with milk, fruit and toast
Yogurt, muffin and fruit
Soup, sandwich with lean meat and milk

A small portion of pasta with tomato sauce
Choose smaller amounts of similar foods if you have less than 2 to 3 hours before an event.

Adapted from Dairy Farmers of Manitoba, Sport Nutrition brochure.

9- DINING OUT

Consider following your personalized meal plan at home for a few weeks before trying it in restaurants. You should become accustomed to serving sizes by measuring the first two times each new food item is eaten. This will train your eye to estimate your portions when you go to restaurants and enable you to stick to your meal plan.

For example, if your plan allows for 3 starches, 2 vegetables, 3 meats or alternatives, 1 fruit and 1 fat with dinner, you could choose ⅔ cup rice plus 1 roll without butter (3 starches), 1 cup salad with ½ cup cooked asparagus (2 vegetables), a fillet of sole (the size of a checkbook = 3 oz meat or alternative), 1 tablespoon of salad dressing on the side (1 fat) and have the fruit later when you get home if it is not offered on the menu. Keep in mind that restaurant portions often exceeds these, so you will have to exercise control in eating the amounts corresponding to your meal plan, then ask for a doggie bag to take the rest home. If you know the restaurant offers huge portions, ask the waiter to put only one half on your plate and the other half in a doggie bag before serving the meal. This will make it easier to resist the urge to finish your plate.

Try to have most meals prepared at home whether you eat them there or at the office. Relying on fast food is not wise. Although some fast food restaurants now offer lower-calorie alternatives, it may be difficult for many people to resist choosing the higher calorie items. It isn't necessarily quicker to go to the drive-through for breakfast. A bagel with low-fat cheese, fruit and yogurt can be picked up more quickly from your kitchen than from a drive-through.

Items to Look for on the Menu

- Baked potato, pasta in tomato or marinara sauce or rice (ask for whole grain), whole grain breads (pita, wraps, bagels)
- Steamed, stir-fried or grilled vegetables or salads with dressing on the side
- Fruit plates, salads or smoothies (made with low-fat milk or yogurt)
- Baked, grilled or steamed fish, lean meats (ex: fillet mignon, sirloin) or tofu, black beans, chickpeas, lentil soups
- Soy milk, low fat (2% **M.F.** or less) milk, yogurt or sherbet

Items to Avoid

- French fries, "poutine" (fries with gravy and cheese), doughnuts, croissants, Alfredo or cream-based pasta sauces
- Deep fried, breaded vegetables, Caesar salad
- Fruit pies and pastries
- Fried chicken or fish, large fatty steaks (ex: rib-eye), deep-fried tofu, refried beans
- Milkshakes and ice cream

Ask merchants to accommodate your requests for whole-grain products (pizza dough, pasta and brown rice) and low fat cheese on pizza, or ask them to use half the usual amount of cheese. The more we request low-fat, low-calorie, high fiber items, the more restaurant owners will be likely to offer them on their menus in order to meet our needs.

10- Body Chemistry & Appetite

Keep in mind that many factors affect appetite. Even the best planner or most motivated dieter will "slip" at times. Premenstrual syndrome (PMS) is one example. PMS is real! It can

> alter metabolic rate, glucose tolerance, appetite, food intake, mood, and behavior...they are seen to be eating an average of 500 calories a day more during the ten days prior to menstruation than during the ten days after—principally from carbohydrates....Many women attempt to restrict their calories...in an effort to control their weight. During the two weeks following menstruation, they may find this relatively easy to do, but during the two weeks before the next menstruation, they may find it hard because they are fighting a natural, hormone-governed increase in **metabolic rate**, appetite, and possibly even a built-in craving for carbohydrate.[15]

Food intake is generally increased after ovulation, during the premenstrual phase, compared with ovulation or the **folliculary phase** of a woman's cycle. The phases of the menstrual cycle were compared in 30 studies with 37 groups. An increased caloric intake during the premenstrual phase compared to the folliculary phase was reported in 25 studies.

One hypothesis is that a temporary **insulin resistance** occurs whereby **insulin** is less efficient at transporting glucose (carbohydrate) into the cell where it can be burned as fuel.

At least 16 neuropeptides and neurotransmitters are known to affect appetite and/or energy expenditure. **Leptin** decreases appetite whereas **ghrelin** increases it. **Leptin** is increased when high-carbohydrate, low-fat meals are eaten, and **ghrelin** is decreased when carbohydrates and **psyllium** fiber (as in Bran Buds™ cereal) are eaten.

Some believe that a deficiency in **serotonin** (another neurotransmitter) is to blame, which could explain sweet cravings. Carbohydrates increase serotonin supply to the brain resulting in a calmer, relieved feeling.

Food & Mood

Nutrition, Concepts and Controversies 5ᵗʰ edition, describes the influence of mood on eating. I could not have worded this better myself.

> The brain has its own survival at stake in directing the body when and what to eat. It is encased in the skull, a hard, inelastic helmet, for its own protection and so cannot expand and contract as can, say, the liver or adipose (fat) tissue. It cannot store its own reserve energy supply in glycogen, fat, or other molecules because those molecules take up space, and it cannot store oxygen with which to oxidize ("burn") those fuels. Therefore the brain must depend on the passing blood supply for its oxygen and fuels...its need for those substances are extraordinary. It comprises only 2 percent of the adult body weight, but at any given time the brain contains 15 percent of the body's blood, and it devours 20 to 30 percent of the fuels that support the **basal metabolism**. Its rapid **metabolism** makes its temperature a degree higher than that of the rest

of the body. Should the blood deliver too little oxygen or **glucose** (carbohydrate), coma would occur within minutes....

The brain is also extremely sensitive to fluctuations in its internal chemical composition. To protect itself from them, it has its own molecular sieve through which the blood must pass.... The blood vessels...are lined with highly selective cells. These cells form a barrier known as the **blood-brain barrier**, which allows desired constituents to enter the brain tissue while restricting others.... Should body stores be inadequate to supply the amounts needed, indications are that the brain may be able to direct eating to obtain carbohydrate at one time and protein at another, depending on its needs.... Thus the food a person eats can influence the brain chemistry by producing high or low concentrations of the precursor nutrients...the nerve cells respond...**serotonin** made from its precursor, the amino acid tryptophan...normally, whole proteins containing tryptophan are eaten...; some other large amino acids in the proteins compete with tryptophan for entry into the brain because they use the same transport mechanism to get across the blood-brain barrier. In this situation tryptophan fails to enter the brain in increased quantities and so does not effectively enhance brain serotonin synthesis. If carbohydrate is fed along with protein, however, it can "help" the protein to deliver tryptophan to the brain because it elicits the secretion of the hormone **insulin**. Insulin drives the other amino acids, but not tryptophan, into body cells, leaving the tryptophan free to enter the brain without competition. Thus, paradoxically, a meal high in carbohydrate, but not one high in protein, eases tryptophan's transport into the brain and so promotes serotonon synthesis...

According to one theory, a high carbohydrate meal raises their brain serotonin, makes them feel good, and so reduces their need for carbohydrates. They therefore eat more protein at the next meal. A high-protein meal creates a serotonin deficit, a loss of the good feeling, and therefore a craving for carbohydrate...it seems to account for what is observed to happen often with weight-control diets. The harder dieters try to restrict carbohydrate the more they seem to crave it. The effect is accentuated if they are **insulin resistant**, as is likely if they are obese. When an **insulin-resistant** person eats carbohydrate, insulin's normal actions do not follow. The person's cells continue to be hungry for glucose (carbohydrate); furthermore, brain **serotonin** does not rise, and so the carbohydrate craving is intensified.... The theory also helps explain why some people describe themselves as anxious, tense, and depressed before eating carbohydrate and peaceful or relaxed afterwards.... This does not mean that people should dose themselves with tryptophan.... An excess of any one (amino acids) could cause deficiencies of others...carbohydrate and protein intakes affect not only insulin secretion but also the secretion of insulin's opposing hormone, glucagon, and glucagon influences the synthesis of neurotransmitters too.... Other hormones that affect the brain — or that are synthesized inside the brain — after eating.... Carbohydrate or tryptophan can also induce fatigue or sleepiness.... Brain serotonin may reduce aggression too....

Men and women may react differently to carbohydrates. A high-carbohydrate meal makes women sleepier and men calmer. Sugar, especially, makes women sleepy. Perhaps this is because women secrete more estrogen hormones than men. Estrogen can reduce serotonin synthesis in the brain, may favor a higher ratio of blood tryptophan to its competing amino acids, and may increase the number of serotonin receptors in the brain. The monthly fluctuation of estrogen secretion may make women react differently to carbohydrate at different times of the month — women's appetites for carbohydrate are keener during the ten days prior to menstruation than during the ten days after.[15]

All the more reason not to skip meals or snacks, get plenty of rest, exercise and limit salt and caffeine.

Supplementation of calcium and magnesium are showing promise. Calcium has been shown to be effective in reducing PMS symptoms at levels of 1200 to 1600 mg per day. Keep in mind that each cup of milk, yogurt or calcium-fortified orange juice provides approximately 300 mg of calcium per serving; most cheeses provide 150 to 200 mg of calcium per 30 g (1 oz).

If you eat on average 2 cups of milk and 2 oz cheese per day, 300 to 500 mg in the form of a supplement could suffice. It can take more than one menstrual cycle before noticing improvements in mood. Although 400 mg of vitamin E taken during the **luteal phase** (second half of the menstrual cycle) has been shown to improve emotional symptoms, risks are also associated with taking this fat-soluble vitamin.

Other nutrients that might be effective include magnesium at levels of 400 to 800 mg/day, cutting out caffeine as well as an intake of 50 to 100 mg of vitamin B_6. More studies are needed of magnesium and vitamin B_6 to support their use.

Go with the Flow

It helps to be aware that PMS affects appetite and cravings. Don't be too hard on yourself if you find it difficult to stick to your meal plan at this time. Don't skip meals or snacks. Avoid high sodium foods and limit caffeine and alcohol as much as possible. Choose more foods from the high-satiety and low-caloric density lists, and remind yourself that your appetite will likely decrease once menstruation begins. Keep exercising; it will help compensate for some extra portions eaten during this time.

Don't be too hard on yourself. Accept the fact that appetite will fluctuate for various reasons. Try the tips described in order to manage your fluctuating appetite as best you can.

CONCLUSION

I hope the information on individual portion needs, balanced meals and snacks, appetite, high satiety foods and caloric density reaches and helps as many people as possible. May they be freed from a struggle of unnecessary hunger and deprivation. Whether their goal is to lose or maintain their current weight, may it set them straight on healthy, balanced eating behaviors and help dispel the myth that one needs to starve in order to lose weight. I believe you can have your cake and eat it too. Just chose a lower calorie cake most of the time.

Remember that your personalized meal plan is meant as a learning tool. Your can eventually put it aside when you have grasped how eating a balanced diet of moderate portions at regular intervals makes you feel, and when you remember what your portion sizes look like.

If you retain one message from this book, let it be: "If you are hungry, by all means, EAT!"

If you are hungry, by all mean, EAT!

REFERENCES

1. *Am J of Obstet Gynecol,* vol 188, #5 (suppl). Girman A, Lee R, Kligler B. An Integrative Medicine Approach to Premenstrual Syndrome. S56-65. May 2003. Permission from Elsevier.

2. American Society for Parenteral and Enteral Nutrition. The Science and Practice of Nutrition Support. A Case-Based Core Curriculum. Kendall/Hunt Publishing Company. Dubuque, Iowa. 2001. Chapter 3.

3. Baribeau, H. Le syndrome prémenstrual: le point sur l'efficacité des médecines alternatives et complémentaires. *Nutrition—science en évolution.* Ordre professionnel des diététistes du Québec, automne 2004. Vol. 2, numéro 2.

4. Biochemistry 1st edition by Campbell. © 1991. p. 510-511. Reprinted with permission of Brooks/Cole, a division of Thomson Learning: www.thomsonrights.com. Fax 800 730-2215

5. Blumberg S. Should Hypoglycemia Patients Be Prescribed a High-Protein Diet? *J Am Diet Assoc.* 2005. 105, no 2:196-197.

6. Canadian Diabetes Association. Lignes directrices de pratique clinique 2003 de l'Association canadienne du diabète pour la prévention et le traitement du diabète au Canada. *Canadian Journal of Diabetes.* Déc. 2003. Vol. 27, suppl. 2.

7. Dairy Farmers of Manitoba, Sport Nutrition brochure.

8. Drummond S, Dixon K, Griffin J, De Looy A. Weight loss on an energy-restricted, low-fat, sugar-containing

diet in overweight sedentary men. *Int J Food Sci Nutr* 2004; 55:279-90.

9. Gélina, MD, Dubost-Bélair, M, Bernier, P et coll. Manuel de nutrition clinique. 2e edition Montréal, Ordre Professionel des diététistes du Québec, 1991. Jacobs-Starkey, L, Gobeil, C, Poliquin, M, Corriveau-Rochon, G, Sainte-Croix, F, Tremblay. S. Hypoglycémie réactionnelle idiopathique. P 6.3-1-2.

10. Larson Duyff, R, MS, RD, FADA, CFCS. American Dietetic Association Complete Food and Nutrition Guide, 2nd edition. John Wiley & Sons, Inc. 2002

11. Lightfoot, Claire, RD, Med, CDE, Pytka, Evelyne S. PDt, BSc, CDE. Making Carbs Count: Advanced Carbohydrate Counting for Intensive Diabetes Management. Canadian Diabetes Association Meeting, Oct. 2004.

12. Macmillan Publishers Ltd: *European Journal of Clinical Nutrition.* S.H.A. Holt, J.C. Brand Miller, P. Petocz, and E. Farmakalidis: A Satiety Index of Common Foods. Table 4. 49: 9; 675-690 (1995).

13. Martin, CL, MS, RN, CDE, White, NH, M.D. National Diabetes Information Clearinghouse. Hypoglycemia in People Who Do Not Have Diabetes. NIH Publication No. 03-3926. March 2003.

14. Messina, V, MPH, RD. The Challenge of Defining Optimal Fat Intake. *Issues in Vegetarian Dietetics.* *Vegetarian Nutrition,* a practice group of the American Dietetic Association. Summer 1998. Volume VII, Number 4.

15. Nutrition, Concepts and Controversies 5th edition by Hamilton/ Whitney/ Sizer. 1991. Reprinted with permission of Brooks/Cole, a division of Thomson Learning: www.thomsonrights.com. Fax 800 730-2215.

16. One Touch® Ultra ® Test strip Insert AW06052707 Revision C.

17. Orr J, Davy B, PhD, RD. Dietary Influences on Peripheral Hormones Regulating Energy Intake: Potential Applications for Weight Management. *J Am Diet Ass.* July 2005. Vol. 105; no 7. 1115-1121.

18. Pike, RL, Brown, ML. Nutrition, an Integrated Approach, Third Edition, Macmillan Publishing Company, New York. 1984. 209-210.

19. Rolls, BJ, PhD, Drewnowski A PhD, Ledikwe JH, PhD. Changing the Energy Density of the Diet as a Strategy for Weight Management. Supplement to *J Am Diet Ass.* May 2005. S98-S103.

20. Service, FJ. Hypoglycemic disorders. Review Article. *N Engl J Med,* 1995 332(17): 1144.

21. United States Department of Agriculture, Center for Nutrition Policy and Promotion. MyPyramid. Food Intake Pattern Calorie Levels. April 2005. CNPP-XX.

22. Vander AJ, M.D., Sherman JH, Ph.D., Luciano DS, Ph.D. Physiologie Humaine 2ème édition. McGraw-Hill, Montréal 1989.

Most people are not taught how to eat, but rather develop eating habits by imitating others.

Appendix 1- Canada's Food Guide

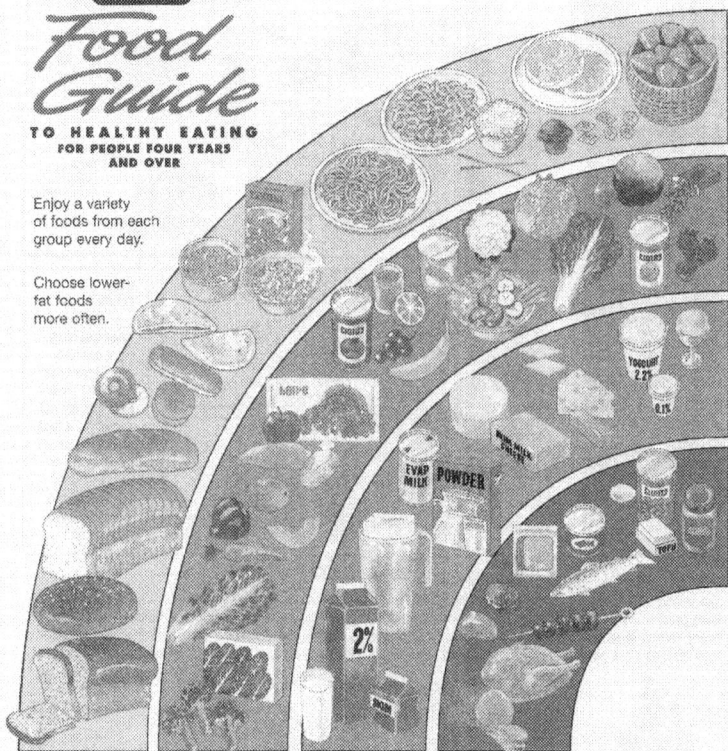

Health Canada / Santé Canada

CANADA'S Food Guide

TO HEALTHY EATING
FOR PEOPLE FOUR YEARS
AND OVER

Enjoy a variety of foods from each group every day.

Choose lower-fat foods more often.

Grain Products
Choose whole grain and enriched products more often.

Vegetables and Fruit
Choose dark green and orange vegetables and orange fruit more often.

Milk Products
Choose lower-fat milk products more often.

Meat and Alternatives
Choose leaner meats, poultry and fish, as well as dried peas, beans and lentils more often.

Canada

Grain Products
5-12
SERVINGS PER DAY

1 Serving — Cold Cereal, 1 Slice, 30 g; Hot Cereal 175 mL, 3/4 cup; 1 Bagel, Pita or Bun
2 Servings — Pasta or Rice 250 mL, 1 cup

Vegetables and Fruit
5-10
SERVINGS PER DAY

1 Serving — 1 Medium Size Vegetable or Fruit; Fresh, Frozen or Canned Vegetables or Fruit 125 mL, 1/2 cup; Salad 250 mL, 1 cup; Juice 125 mL, 1/2 cup

Milk Products
SERVINGS PER DAY
Children 4-9 years: 2-3
Youth 10-16 years: 3-4
Adults: 2-4
Pregnant and Breast-feeding Women: 3-4

1 Serving — Milk 250 mL, 1 cup; Cheese 3"x1"x1", 50 g; 2 Slices 50 g; Yogurt 175 g, 3/4 cup

Other Foods

Taste and enjoyment can also come from other foods and beverages that are not part of the 4 food groups. Some of these foods are higher in fat or Calories, so use these foods in moderation.

Meat and Alternatives
2-3
SERVINGS PER DAY

1 Serving — Meat, Poultry or Fish 50-100 g; Fish; Beans 125-250 mL; 1/3-2/3 Can 50-100 g; 1-2 Eggs; Tofu 100 g; Peanut Butter 30 mL, 2 tbsp, 1/3 cup

Different People Need Different Amounts of Food
The amount of food you need every day from the 4 food groups and other foods depends on your age, body size, activity level, whether you are male or female and if you are pregnant or breast-feeding. That's why the Food Guide gives a lower and higher number of servings for each food group. For example, young children can choose the lower number of servings, while male teenagers can go to the higher number. Most other people can choose servings somewhere in between.

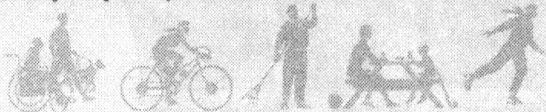

Consult *Canada's Physical Activity Guide to Healthy Active Living* to help you build physical activity into your daily life.

Enjoy eating well, being active and feeling good about yourself. That's VITALITY

© Minister of Public Works and Government Services Canada, 1997
Cat. No. H39-252/1992E   ISBN 0-662-19648-1
No changes permitted. Reprint permission not required.

Appendix 2- Revisions to the 2005 Dietary Guidelines

Physical activity: at least 30 minutes/day of moderate-to-vigorous exercise;
60 minutes/day to prevent weight gain in most adults;
60-90 minutes/day for weight loss.

Fruit and vegetables: 9 servings/day

Fats: 20-35 % of calories provided form fat, most unsaturated fat;
A maximum of 10% of calories from saturated fat.

Carbohydrates: Choose and prepare foods and beverages with little added sugar.

Milk: Consume 3 cups of skim or low-fat milk or milk products each day

Salt: Avoid consuming more than 2300 mg of sodium per day. A low-sodium product is considered to contain 140 mg of sodium or less per serving.

Think of learning your estimated caloric needs and food portions as homework that may teach you how much food to eat in a day in order to maintain or lose weight. Once learned, the meal plan may be set aside, only to be referred to occasionally to refresh your memory.

GLOSSARY OF TERMS

Adipose tissue: fat tissue in the body.

Adjusted body weight: an estimation of metabolically active weight in the obese. Calculating estimated calorie needs using the actual weight of an obese person would over-estimate their needs because fat tissue is not very metabolically active (does not burn many calories).

Autonomic symptoms: symptoms generated by the autonomic nervous system which transmits nervous impulses to organs and glands "automatically", hence without out intentional control.

Basal energy expenditure (or metabolic rate): the amount of calories (energy) one burns at complete rest (after awakening and fasting for 12 to 14 hours). Age, gender and amount of lean tissue affect basal metabolic rate.

Blood-brain barrier: made up of cells in the blood vessels communicating with the brain which selectively "let in" or "block out" compounds.

Body Mass Index (BMI): weight in kilograms (kg) divided by height in meters squared. A tool used to measure obesity.

Calories (kilocalories or kcal): a unit of energy; the amount of heat needed to raise the temperature of one kilogram (kg) of water by 1 Celsius degree.

Carbohydrate: a source of food energy in the form of simple sugars, starches, fruit and dairy products.

Relatively small amounts are contained in vegetables. Glucose is its simplest form. Fiber is an indigestible form of carbohydrate.

Carbohydrate-choice: a starch or grain product, fruit or dairy portion from the food group exchanges lists.

Concentrated sweets: include table sugar, brown sugar, honey, syrup, molasses, fructose, or foods such as desserts prepared with these ingredients in concentrated amounts.

Desirable body weight: a "healthy body weight"; usually corresponding to a BMI of 18.5 to 25. A BMI of 27 is acceptable in the elderly. There are exceptions such as very muscular people who may have a BMI over 25 yet still be at a healthy weight with a low percentage of body fat.

Dairy products: includes milk and yogurt. Although cheese is a dairy product, count it as a meat alternative in this program (refer to the Food Exchange lists).

DHA: an omega-3 fatty acid made from linolenic acid in fish.

Diabetes: an illness whereby the pancreas does not produce enough insulin to lower blood sugar within a normal range.

EPA: an omega-3 fatty acid made from linolenic acid in fish.

Essential fatty acids: fatty acids we must get from our diet. Our bodies cannot produce sufficient amounts to meet our needs. These are linoleic (an omega-6 fatty acid) acid and linolenic acid (an omega-3 fatty acid).

Exchanges (food exchanges): a portion size or one food choice in a given food group.

Fat choice: added fat portion listed among the food exchanges such as oil, salad dressing, peanut-butter, seeds, avocado and olives.

Fermentation: the chemical decomposition of foods in the intestine with the formation of gas.

Fiber: an indigestible carbohydrate.
> **Insoluble fiber:** wheat, rice and corn bran are examples.
> **Soluble fiber:** guar gum, pectin, oat and barley bran are examples.

Folliculary phase: the phase of the menstrual cycle when an ovary develops until maturity prior to ovulation.

Food journal: a daily record of food intake and meal times.

Ghrelin: an appetite enhancing hormone; levels decrease with carbohydrate and psyllium ingestion; dietary protein shows conflicting effects on ghrelin.

Glucagon: insulin's counter-regulatory hormone. Glucagon helps drive glucose (sugar) into the bloodstream.

Gluconeogenesis: the conversion of non-carbohydrates (such as amino acids) to glucose (carbohydrate).

Glucose: the simplest form of carbohydrate (one molecule).

Glucose intolerance: a condition of elevated blood sugar levels not high enough to be considered Diabetes.

Glycogen: carbohydrate reserves in the liver and muscles.

Harris Benedict Equation: an equation used to estimate caloric needs of an individual.

High satiety foods: foods that increase satiety (the absence of hunger).

Hypoglycemia: blood sugar below normal range. Symptoms include hunger, irritability, trouble concentrating, anxiety, fatigue, headaches, weakness, sweating, dizziness, trembling, heart palpitations, blurred vision and loss of consciousness. Confusion or strange behavior such as trouble speaking and lack of coordination may also occur.

> **Fasting hypoglycemia:** occurs after fasting, between meals or after exercising.
>
> **Reactive hypoglycemia:** occurs within four hour of eating.

Hydrogenated: oils that are transformed to be solid at room temperature such as shortening.

Insulin: a hormone that drives glucose (sugar) from the bloodstream into cells.

Insulin resistance: a condition whereby insulin is less effective at driving glucose (sugar) into the cells of the body.

Ketone bodies: "the product of the incomplete breakdown of fat when carbohydrate is not available."[15]

Ketosis: "an undesirably high concentration of ketone bodies, such as acetone, in the blood and urine." [15]

Legumes: dried bean, lentils, chickpeas, split peas, are examples.

Leptin: an appetite suppressing hormone; levels increase when high-carbohydrate low-fat meals are eaten compared with low-carbohydrate meals.

Low blood sugar: blood sugar below normal range.

Low-carbohydrate diet: a diet that does not provide most of its calories from carbohydrates.

Low energy density: foods of relatively low caloric density per weight.

Luteal phase: second half of the menstrual cycle.

Metabolic rate (basal): the rate at which the body burns calories to perform its involuntary bodily functions such as circulation, respiration and tissue repair.

% M.F.: the percentage by weight of a food consisting of milk fat.

Monounsaturated fats: fats that lower levels of the "lousy" LDL-cholesterol carriers without lowering levels of the "healthy" HDL-cholesterol carriers. They include olive oil, canola oil, peanuts and avocado.

Personalized meal plan: a planned number of portions per day and their distribution in meals and snacks corresponding to the caloric needs of an individual.

Polyunsaturated fats: fats that lower levels of the "healthy" HDL-cholesterol carriers while lowering levels of the "lousy" LDL-cholesterol carriers. They include safflower oil, sunflower seed oil and corn oil. Omega-3 unsaturated fats promote heart health by lowering triglyceride levels, blood pressure and reducing the risk of blood clots and arrhythmia.

Protein choice: a meat or alternative exchange (meat, fish, poultry, egg, cheese, legumes such as lentils, chickpeas, etc.). One may have more than one choice or exchange of a given food group per meal or snack.

Psyllium: a seed from India containing a rich content of soluble fiber known to slow carbohydrate absorption, and lower blood cholesterol.

Registered Dietitian: a professional with the required credentials in his or her province, state or country to legally practice the profession of dietetics or nutrition. Also called a Dietitian or Nutritionist. A Bachelor's degree and internship are usually required.

Satiety: the absence of hunger between meals/snacks. "The feeling of fullness or satisfaction after a meal."[15]

Saturated fat: fats that are solid at room temperature such as butter, meat fat, bacon, cheese and milk fat. Although hydrogenated fats are solid at room temperature, technically they are not classified as saturated although they are just as harmful, or even worse; they are made from liquid oil that is transformed into a solid such as shortening.

Serotonin: a brain neurotransmitter affected by carbohydrate intake.

Simple sugars: short-chain carbohydrates such as table sugar, brown sugar, syrup, molasses and honey.

Soluble fiber: a fiber known to slow carbohydrate absorption, and lower blood cholesterol. Oat bran, barley legumes and guar gum (Benefiber™) are examples of rich sources.

Sodium: the fraction of salt associated with fluid retention and blood pressure elevation in sodium sensitive individuals.

Starch: long-chain carbohydrates such as in flour, rice, corn, potatoes and beans.

Sugar alcohols: sweeteners that contain fewer calories than sugar and do not promote tooth decay. Over consumption can cause diarrhea in certain individual. They include xylitol, maltitol, sorbitol and polydextrose.

AAB Publishing Quick Order Form

Fax orders: 514-937-2626. Send this form.

Website orders: www.aabpublishing.com

Telephone orders: 1-866-342-9313 toll-free.

E-mail orders: orders@aabpublishing.com

Postal orders: AAB Publishing PO Box 563-A, Station H, Montreal, QC H3G 2L5, Canada

Please send number of copy(ies): ___ of Eat Often, Feel Great & Lose Weight.

Name: _____

Address: _____

City: _____ Province/State: _____

Postal/Zip Code: _____Telephone: _____

E-mail address: _____

Price: $24.95 (USD)
Sales tax: Please add sales tax and GST for products shipped to Quebec.

Shipping by air
Canada: $4.00 (CND) for the first book. Add $2.00 for each additional book.
International: $9.00 (USD) for the first book. Add $5.00 for each additional book.
Total payment: _____

Payment: Cheque   Credit card:
                Visa   MasterCard

Card number: _____

Name on card: _____

Exp. date: _____